Raymond M. Costello, Ph. D.
Department of Psychiatry
University of Texas
Medical School at San Antonio
7703 Floyd Curl Drive
San Antonio, Texas  78229

# Pharmacotherapy and Psychotherapy: Paradoxes Problems and Progress

*Formulated by the*
*Committee on Research*

Group for the Advancement of Psychiatry

BRUNNER/MAZEL *Publishers* ● New York

This publication was produced for the Group for the Advancement of Psychiatry by the Mental Health Materials Center, Inc., New York.

*International Standard Book Number 87630-114-6 clothbound*

*Library of Congress Catalog Card Number 75-6951*

*Printed in the United States of America*

BRUNNER/MAZEL, Inc.
64 University Place, New York, N. Y. 10003

# TABLE OF CONTENTS

# STATEMENT OF PURPOSE

THE GROUP FOR THE ADVANCEMENT OF PSYCHIATRY has a membership of approximately 300 psychiatrists, most of whom are organized in the form of a number of working committees. These committees direct their efforts toward the study of various aspects of psychiatry and the application of this knowledge to the fields of mental health and human relations.

Collaboration with specialists in other disciplines has been and is one of GAP's working principles. Since the formation of GAP in 1946 its members have worked closely with such other specialists as anthropologists, biologists, economists, statisticians, educators, lawyers, nurses, psychologists, sociologists, social workers, and experts in mass communication, philosophy, and semantics. GAP envisages a continuing program of work according to the following aims:

1. To collect and appraise significant data in the fields of psychiatry, mental health, and human relations
2. To reevaluate old concepts and to develop and test new ones
3. To apply the knowledge thus obtained for the promotion of mental health and good human relations

GAP is an independent group, and its reports represent the composite findings and opinions of its members only, guided by its many consultants.

PHARMACOTHERAPY AND PSYCHOTHERAPY: PARADOXES, PROBLEMS AND PROGRESS *was formulated by the Committee on Research, which acknowledges on page 269 the participation of others in the preparation of this report. The members of this committee, as well as other committees and the officers of the GAP, are listed below.*

COMMITTEE ON RESEARCH
Morris A. Lipton, Chapel Hill, Chr.
Stanley H. Eldred, Belmont, Mass.
Louis A. Gottschalk, Irvine, Calif.

Donald F. Klein, Glen Oaks, N.Y.
Gerald L. Klerman, Boston
Ralph R. Notman, Brookline, Mass.
Eberhard H. Uhlenhuth, Chicago

**COMMITTEE ON ADOLESCENCE**
Joseph D. Noshpitz, Washington, Chr.
Maurice R. Friend, New York
Warren J. Gadpaille, Englewood, Colo.
Charles A. Malone, Philadelphia
Silvio J. Onesti, Jr., Belmont, Mass.
Jeanne Spurlock, Silver Spring, Md.
Sidney L. Werkman, Denver

**COMMITTEE ON AGING**
Prescott W. Thompson, San Jose, Chr.
Robert N. Butler, Washington, D.C.
Charles M. Gaitz, Houston
Lawrence F. Greenleigh, Los Angeles
Maurice E. Linden, Philadelphia
Robert D. Patterson, Lexington, Mass.
F. Conyers Thompson, Jr., Atlanta
Jack Weinberg, Chicago

**COMMITTEE ON CHILD PSYCHIATRY**
Joseph M. Green, Tucson, Ariz., Chr.
Paul L. Adams, Miami
E. James Anthony, St. Louis
James M. Bell, Canaan, N.Y.
Harlow Donald Dunton, New York
Joseph Fischoff, Detroit
John F. Kenward, Chicago
Ake Mattsson, Charlottesville
John F. McDermott, Jr., Honolulu
Theodore Shapiro, New York
Exie E. Welsch, New York
Virginia N. Wilking, New York

**COMMITTEE ON THE COLLEGE STUDENT**
Robert L. Arnstein, Hamden, Conn., Chr.
Harrison P. Eddy, New York
Malkah Tolpin Notman, Brookline, Mass.
Gloria C. Onque, Pittsburgh
Kent E. Robinson, Towson, Md.
Earle Silber, Chevy Chase, Md.
Tom G. Stauffer, White Plains, N.Y.

**COMMITTEE ON THE FAMILY**
Joseph Satten, San Francisco, Chr.
C. Christian Beels, Bronx, N.Y.
Ivan Boszormenyi-Nagy, Wyncote, Pa.
Murray Bowen, Chevy Chase
Henry U. Grunebaum, Boston
Margaret M. Lawrence, Pomona, N.Y.
David Mendell, Houston
Carol Nadelson, Boston

Norman L. Paul, Cambridge
Israel Zwerling, Philadelphia

**COMMITTEE ON GOVERNMENTAL AGENCIES**
Sidney S. Goldensohn, Jamaica, N.Y. Chr.
William S. Allerton, Richmond
Albert M. Biele, Philadelphia
Paul Chodoff, Washington, D.C.
John E. Nardini, Washington, D.C.
Donald B. Peterson, Fulton, Mo.
Harvey L. P. Resnik, Chevy Chase, Md.
Harold Rosen, Baltimore
Harvey Lee Ruben, New Haven

**COMMITTEE ON INTERNATIONAL RELATIONS**
Bryant M. Wedge, Washington, D.C., Chr.
Francis F. Barnes, Chevy Chase
Eric A. Baum, Cambridge
Alexander Gralnick, Port Chester, N.Y.
Rita R. Rogers, Torrance, Calif.
Bertram H. Schaffner, New York
Mottram P. Torre, New Orleans
Roy M. Whitman, Cincinnati
Ronald M. Wintrob, Hartford

**COMMITTEE ON MEDICAL EDUCATION**
Saul I. Harrison, Ann Arbor, Chr.
Raymond Feldman, Boulder, Colo.
David R. Hawkins, Charlottesville
Harold I. Lief, Philadelphia
John E. Mack, Chestnut Hill, Mass.
Herbert Pardes, Brooklyn, N.Y.
Robert Alan Senescu, New York
Bryce Templeton, Philadelphia
Paul Tyler Wilson, Bethesda, Md.

**COMMITTEE ON MENTAL HEALTH SERVICES**
W. Walter Menninger, Topeka, Chr.
Allan Beigel, Tucson, Ariz.
Eugene M. Caffey, Jr., Washington, D.C.
Merrill T. Eaton, Omaha
James B. Funkhouser, Richmond, Va.
Robert S. Garber, Belle Mead, N.J.
Stanley Hammons, Frankfort, Ky.
Donald Scherl, Boston
Herzl R. Spiro, Princeton, N.J.
Jack A. Wolford, Pittsburgh

**COMMITTEE ON MENTAL RETARDATION**
Henry H. Work, Washington, D.C., Chr.
Howard V. Bair, Parsons, Kans.
Norman R. Bernstein, Boston

Robert Michels, New York
Andrew P. Morrison, Cambridge
William C. Offenkrantz, Chicago
Franz K. Reichsman, Brooklyn
Lewis L. Robbins, Glen Oaks, N.Y.
Joseph P. Tupin, Sacramento
Herbert Weiner, Bronx, N.Y.

CONTRIBUTING MEMBERS
Carlos C. Alden, Jr., Buffalo
Charlotte G. Babcock, Pittsburgh
Grace Baker, New York
Walter E. Barton, Hartland, Vt.
Spencer Bayles, Houston, Tex.
Anne R. Benjamin, Chicago
Ivan C. Berlien, Coral Gables, Fla.
Sidney Berman, Washington, D.C.
Grete L. Bibring, Cambridge
Carl A. L. Binger, Cambridge
H. Waldo Bird, St. Louis
Wilfred Bloomberg, Boston
H. Keith H. Brodie, Durham, N.C.
Eugene Brody, Baltimore
Matthew Brody, Brooklyn, N.Y.
Ewald W. Busse, Durham
Dale Cameron, Guilford, Conn.
Ian L. W. Clancey, Maitland, Ont., Can.
Sanford I. Cohen, Boston
Robert Coles, Cambridge
Frank J. Curran, New York
William D. Davidson, Washington, D.C.
Leonard J. Duhl, Berkeley
Lloyd C. Elam, Nashville
Joseph T. English, New York
Louis C. English, Pomona, N.Y.
O. Spurgeon English, Narberth, Pa.
Dana L. Farnsworth, Boston
Stuart M. Finch, Tucson, Ariz.
Alfred Flarsheim, Chicago
Archie R. Foley, New York
Alan Frank, Albuquerque, N.M.
Daniel X. Freedman, Chicago
Albert J. Glass, Chicago
Alvin I. Goldfarb, New York
Louis A. Gottschalk, Irvine, Calif.
Milton Greenblatt, Sepulveda, Calif.
Maurice H. Greenhill, Rye, N.Y.
John H. Greist, Indianapolis
Roy R. Grinker, Sr., Chicago
Ernest M. Gruenberg, Poughkeepsie, N.Y.

Edward O. Harper, Cleveland, Ohio
Mary O'Neill Hawkins, New York
J. Cotter Hirschberg, Topeka
Edward J. Hornick, New York
Joseph Hughes, Philadelphia
Portia Bell Hume, Berkeley
Irene M. Josselyn, Phoenix
Jay Katz, New Haven
Sheppard G. Kellam, Chicago
Gerald L. Klerman, Boston
Othilda M. Krug, Cincinnati
Zigmond M. Lebensohn, Washington, D.C.
Henry D. Lederer, Washington, D.C.
Robert L. Leopold, Philadelphia
Alan I. Levenson, Tucson, Ariz.
Earl A. Loomis, New York
Reginald S. Lourie, Washington, D.C.
Alfred O. Ludwig, Boston
Jeptha R. MacFarlane, Westbury, N.Y.
John A. MacLeod, Cincinnati
Sidney G. Margolin, Denver
Peter A. Martin, Southfield, Mich.
Helen V. McLean, Chicago
Jack H. Mendelson, Belmont, Mass.
Karl A. Menninger, Topeka
Eugene Meyer, Baltimore
James G. Miller, Louisville, Ky.
John A. P. Millet, Nyack, N.Y.
Peter B. Neubauer, New York
Rudolph G. Novick, Lincolnwood, Ill.
Lucy D. Ozarin, Bethesda, Md.
Bernard L. Pacella, New York
William L. Peltz, Manchester, Vt.
Irving Philips, San Francisco
Charles A. Pinderhughes, Boston
Eveoleen N. Rexford, Cambridge
Milton Rosenbaum, Bronx, N.Y.
W. Donald Ross, Cincinnati
Lester H. Rudy, Chicago
David S. Sanders, Beverly Hills
Kurt O. Schlesinger, San Francisco
Calvin F. Settlage, Sausalito, Calif.
Richard I. Shader, Newton Centre, Mass.
Harley C. Shands, New York
Albert J. Silverman, Ann Arbor
Benson R. Snyder, Cambridge
John P. Spiegel, Waltham, Mass.
Brandt F. Steele, Denver
Eleanor A. Steele, Denver
Rutherford B. Stevens, New York
Alan A. Stone, Cambridge, Mass.

# COMMITTEE ACKNOWLEDGMENTS

Special thanks are due Sidney Gimpel, who was particularly helpful in the preparation of this report, as a consultant; and to Jack S. Brandes, M.D., Ginsburg Fellow of GAP assigned to the Committee on Research during this period.

Currently, the Committee on Research is working under the chairmanship of Donald F. Klein, M.D., while Morris A. Lipton, M.D., Ph.D., who chaired the Committee during preparation of this report, has remained with the Committee as a member.

# PREFACE

GAP is a quilt of many colors. Its 21 committees and various occasional task forces, stitched together by a loyalty to the organization as a whole, cover a diversity of subjects in their individual deliberations. Over the past thirty years GAP reports have been addressed to a variety of audiences and aims. Clinical practice, research, social issues, education, psychiatry's relations with other disciplines—all have been fuel for the fires of creative thought from which come publications designed to inform, to influence, to reform and to stimulate their readers. Many are now antiquated, composed as they were in response to problems since become matters of mere historical interest. But a few live on, imbued with a scholarship that has made them signal contributions to psychiatry as a scientific discipline.

The volume in hand is destined to become such a work. Its authors, reviewing the scientific studies on the use and effectiveness of psychotherapy and pharmacotherapy, explode the myth that the two are mutually incompatible, show the dangers of an irrational bias toward one or the other, suggest areas and strategies for further research, and point to some of the ethical issues that must be faced in such future investigations. And they do so with an orderliness of presentation and a clarity of prose that make introductory glossing superfluous. The reader is urged to turn the page—*res ipsa loquitur.*

John C. Nemiah, M.D., President
GROUP FOR THE ADVANCEMENT OF PSYCHIATRY

13

# 1

## INTRODUCTION: PROBLEMS OF INTEGRATION

There are at least two generalizations substantiated by the history of medical therapeutics. The first is that the greater the number and variety of treatments employed for a given illness, the greater the likelihood that none of them is definitive or completely effective. The second is that it is not at all unusual to find empirical practice to be totally unrelated to existing theories of disease (e.g., foxglove was used for the treatment of dropsy long before the etiology of edema with heart failure was recognized).

These generalizations seem to be especially relevant in any consideration of the current treatments advocated for mental illness. Psychiatric treatment today may be characterized by intensive, extensive, and frequently expensive commitments to the treatment of a broad range of mental illness. Thus, for psychotic patients there are advocates of nutrition and megavitamins, phenothiazines, butyrophenones and electroconvulsive therapy, intensive and prolonged psychotherapy, supportive and group psychotherapy, and behavioral shaping along the lines of a token economy. For the neuroses, there are available a vast number of minor tranquilizers and an equally large number of forms of psychotherapy. The determinants of the type of treatment offered are hardly ever very clear. To a considerable extent they depend upon the training and ideology of the manpower available for treatment. Those without licenses to use drugs, and who therefore cannot prescribe them, frequently oppose their use. Similarly, those lacking experience with drugs, generally trained before drugs were available, tend to oppose them. Thus, while vigorous

15

arguments continue among adherents of the various schools of psychotherapy, with each proponent emphasizing the theoretical and technical advantages of his school, there remains a consensus that drugs play only a minor role in treatment. Some feel they are contraindicated and perhaps damaging; others use them for symptom relief or as adjuvants to other forms of therapy.

The converse is equally true. Physicians with licenses for the prescribing of drugs—but who lack knowledge of psychotherapeutic principles and practice and who are indeed often suspicious of them—tend to use drugs, frequently in inappropriate dosages and occasionally to the detriment of the patient. Even among those who are reasonably well trained in both pharmacotherapy and psychotherapy, and who feel comfortable using them, there is a conspicuous lack of reasoned comprehension for their joint use, and especially for their interaction.

Nor has the matter of timing the administration of either form of treatment been adequately researched. The argument for drugs versus psychotherapy or psychotherapy versus drugs or even for their conjoint use is somewhat naïve. It is likely that there are conditions in which drugs may be needed for the initiation of treatment but may be discontinued while psychotherapy continues. It is equally likely that drugs may be useful intermittently during the course of psychotherapy. Finally, there may well be periods when psychotherapy should or must be interrupted or discontinued while drug therapy is maintained. It is likely that in practice all these conditions occur, but research data on them are sorely lacking.

To a considerable extent, physicians who have been exposed to the theory and practice of psychotherapy and also of pharmacotherapy behave like a split-brain preparation. We have learned much about psychogenic etiology, and about a variety of forms of psychotherapy. We have also learned a good deal about the use of drugs for specific illnesses (or certainly for symptoms) and have at least a rudimentary notion about the pharmacological mode of action of the drugs. However, the translation of psychological conflict into cellular malfunction, or the reverse translation of disordered biochemical mechanisms into pathological behavior, is still beyond us. Hence, while we may be reasonably comfortable within either frame of reference taken separately, in those complex therapeutic tasks requiring both frames of reference we lack a coherent body of theory or even integrating hypotheses which might combine the insights drawn from psychodynamic observation and investigation with those coming from the more recent neuropsychopharmacological treatments.

The split-brain preparation is able to perform adequately tasks which have been learned with each hemisphere. But when complex tasks requiring both hemispheres are required, the two hemispheres may compete, with resulting confusion of cognition and performance. The situation may not be dissimilar in the relations between pharmacotherapy and psychotherapy, with resulting misuse of both.

## Psychopharmacological drugs today

In the fifteen years since pharmacotherapy has become a major influence and procedure in the theory and treatment of mental or emotional illness, it has burgeoned into a scientific enterprise involving many hundreds of workers and resulting in the publication of more than 10,000 papers ranging in scope from the molecular action of the psychotropic drugs on specific enzyme systems to their clinical efficacy in various types of illness. Several textbooks of psychopharmacology have appeared.

Psychopharmacological drugs have also become a major component of the drug industry. Levine[1] estimated that more than 178,000,000 prescriptions for psychotropic drugs were written in 1967 in the United States.* About 17% of all prescriptions written were for drugs of this type. The patient cost was $692,000,000. Chlordiazepoxide proved to be the single most popular prescription, with patient costs of almost $150,000,000. If drug combinations in which psychotropic drugs are combined with antispasmodics or vasodilators and the like are added to this total, probably 25% of all prescriptions contain psychotropic drugs. The distribution of prescriptions is as follows:

| | |
|---|---|
| Major tranquilizers (phenothiazines) | 9.5% |
| Minor tranquilizers (anti-anxiety agents) | 34.4% |
| Antidepressants (tricyclics) | 8.6% |
| Amphetamines | 15.4% |
| Sedatives (barbiturates) | 12.9% |
| Hypnotics (for insomnia) | 19.2% |

Other data pertinent to usage reveal that the heaviest drug users are in the age group 40-59 and that 70% of all psychotropic drug prescriptions are written by general practitioners, gynecologists, internists and surgeons, although psychiatrists and neurologists as a specialty group prescribe them at a greater rate than any other M.D. specialty.

A survey of the use of psychotropic drugs in California[2] gives similar results. Frequent use of psychotropic drugs is reported by 17% of the adults sampled and is almost twice as high in women as in men. Among men, stimulants are used most commonly in the 30-year age group, tranquilizers in the 40's and 50's, and sedatives from age 60 on. About 30% of a random sample had used a psychotropic drug in the preceding 12 months.

Figures such as these are impressive because they indicate a

* See H. C. Lennard *et al.* MYSTIFICATION AND DRUG MISUSE (New York: Harper & Row, 1971) page vii. Lennard and co-workers reported that the figure was 202,000,000 in 1970, and there is every reason to believe that this figure has continued to escalate.

very high incidence of emotional distress in the population at large. They also suggest that there is a low tolerance of this type of distress and that other solutions for it leave much to be desired, because they are either unavailable or relatively ineffective. Of course, it is also possible that a substantial portion of this high use rate does, in fact, represent transient use of drugs.

A proper estimate of the incidence of drug use for the solution of emotional problems should add to the figures cited here nonprescription items like the antihistamines, which are sold for relief of insomnia and tension states, and drugs like alcohol, marijuana and opiates, the use of which is also rapidly increasing. It is difficult to obtain adequate data on the incidence of usage of nonprescription and illegal drugs in the population, but the evidence is quite clear that it is high and is not declining.

Although the use of psychotropic drugs is astonishingly great and the industry certainly a major one, so too is what might be called "the psychotherapy industry." Here it is difficult to obtain precise data, but there are approximately 2,000 mental health clinics in which full-time psychiatrists represent about 5% of the professional personnel, and full and part-time psychiatrists represent about 25% of total personnel. About 15,000 mental health workers employed in these clinics are clinical psychologists, social workers or other types of professionals who are unable to prescribe drugs and have little or no training in their use and utility. In addition, we may estimate that about 15,000 psychiatrists in the United States are performing psychotherapy about half the time. Simple calculation reveals that this professional time amounts to approximately 300,000 psychotherapeutic hours a week, or more than 10,000,000 hours per year performed by psychiatrists. At a conservative estimate, this would represent an industry of about $250,000,000 annually. If one adds to this psychotherapy by clinical psychologists, social workers, marriage counselors and others, it would appear reasonable to double the dollar value of this industry. The cost of community mental health centers alone is estimated at $223,600,000 annually. It therefore seems reasonable to estimate that the size of "the psychotherapy industry" is at least of an order of magnitude comparable to that of the pharmacotherapy industry. Large numbers of psychiatrists and other mental health workers are involved, and large numbers of patients are seen. Curiously, at this date, there is substantially less research going on in the area of psychotherapy than there is in psychopharmacology.

## Current attitudes toward psychoactive drugs

If these data are sufficiently reliable to be taken seriously, we are immediately struck by a series of paradoxes. Historically, the reception of psychotropic drugs by the advocates of psychogenic etiology and psychotherapeutic treatment was far from cordial. Psychotherapeutic drugs were called chemical straitjackets, which treated society rather than patients. They were considered to be suppressors of symptoms that mask the progress of the illness, which might otherwise be more readily corrected with proper psychotherapy. Many felt that because these drugs reduced symptoms and could generate magical transference qualities to drugs, they would actually be impediments to some more etiologically related form of therapy, that is, psychotherapy. Most psychotherapists tended to ignore their existence and rarely made reference to them. Thus, nearly a decade ago, Whitman[3] pointed out that the psychoanalytic literature contained no references to psychotropic drugs. This situation has remained essentially unchanged. Although some psychoanalysts have done research with drugs, the results have not seemed appropriate to the publication policies of the psychoanalytic journals, and these workers publish in other types of journals. Psychoanalysts apparently do use psychotropic drugs, but as a rule reluctantly and to an unknown but presumably limited extent (see Chapter 6).

On the other hand, to many nonpsychiatrists and to organically minded psychiatrists, drugs were initially visualized as panaceas which by their therapeutic effectiveness proved the organic nature of mental illness, disproved psychogenic theories of etiology, and rendered the "talking therapies" unnecessary.

As mentioned earlier on, even the most eclectic psychiatrists who use both psychotherapy and psychotropic drugs do so with no real theory or integrated rationale for such combined therapy. The question may then be asked why this is so. To answer it, one must pose a series of prior questions: whether these treatment modalities interact; if so, how they interact; and whether they are additive, synergistic or detrimental to each other. These are research questions, and it is surprising to see how little systematic work has been done in this area. It may therefore be proper to inquire into the reasons.

One of the primary reasons has to do with competing theories or ideological rationales (see discussion of "prototheories" in Chapter 4) of the etiology or pathogenesis of mental illness. Altogether too often these viewpoints are treated as being mutually exclusive. Thus, it is difficult to offer a rationale for the use of tricyclic antidepressent chemicals to those who take a dynamically oriented position like that reflected in the formulation of depression as the result of conflict between ego and superego in individuals who have failed to develop these functions adequately because of disturbed interpersonal relationships during childhood. Rather, the dynamically oriented therapists strive through psychotherapeutic contacts to resolve the conflicts, permit the patient's growth and maturation, and thus achieve a true cure. Similar arguments can be and have been made for the etiology and hence the treatment of schizophrenia and the neuroses. According to this rationale, these illnesses are considered psychogenic in origin and thus require psychotherapy for cure, leaving no place for pharmacological agents.

On the other hand, those who view depression as an illness with a genetic component characterized by diminution of central biogenic amines, or of the sensitivity of central receptors, consider the use of somatic therapies designed to restore the biogenic amines to an appropriate functional state to be rational, and psychotherapy secondary or perhaps irrelevant. Again, if schizophrenia is viewed as an illness with a significant genetic component, characterized by a state of hypervigilance and CNS instability, the use of receptor-blocking agents like the phenothiazines is rational and the role of psychotherapy is minimal.

The tendency toward exclusiveness and competition in ideology, though common, is unfortunate. Few would deny in principle that psychogenesis may have material consequences (like alteration in metabolic function). Equally, not all genotypes express themselves as phenotypes; an appropriate environment is required for genetic expression. Thus, there is no rational reason why psychogenic illnesses should not be treated somatically, nor why somatic illnesses might not benefit from psychological intervention. Yet, the tendency to polarize is strong and persistent.

Such polarization can only be diminished by the accumulation of empirical evidence that pharmacological treatment of psychogenically induced illnesses is indeed possible. McKinney et al[4] have shown this to be the case with monkeys in whom seriously disturbed behavior is induced by psychological stress. McKinney finds that rehabilitation of such monkeys can be achieved psychologically, using "monkey therapists." It can also be achieved pharmacologically with chlorpromazine therapy.* Such animal paradigms may go far in reducing the

---

* Similar findings have been reported by Corson et al, who found that certain dogs, which could not tolerate a Pavlovian harness for conditioning or which were aggressive and violent, failed to respond to meprobamate or phenothiazines but did

ideological conflict between psychotherapists and pharmacotherapists.

Concepts of etiology invariably carry with them implications for concepts of optimal treatment because cure in the
fullest sense of the word can be achieved only by removal or
correction of the etiologic agent and its sequential reverbera-
tions. Treatment that does not eliminate the etiologic agent is
at best symptomatic and may be only palliative or even harmful. Yet most treatment, especially of chronic ills in medical or
surgical practice, is of this order.

## Concepts of cure in treatment of mental illness

Something should perhaps be said about the concept of cure
in the treatment of mental illness. In medicine, *treatment*, a
loosely used term, can be structured in a hierarchy as follows:

OUTCOMES OF THERAPY
1—Total Reversal, Future Prevention, No Residue
2—Total Reversal, Future Prevention, Residue
3—Total Reversal, No Future Prevention, No Residue
4—Total Reversal, No Future Prevention, Residue
5—Symptomatic Reversal with Spontaneous Healing
6—Total Reversal, with Continued Therapy
7—Partial Arrest, with Slowing of Progress
8—No Arrest, with Symptom Relief
9—No Benefit
10—Harm

respond to amphetamines in the "paradoxical" fashion of hyperkinetic children.
(See: S. Corson *et al*, in "Proceedings of an International Symposium on the Rele-
vance of Animal Psychopathological Model to the Human," sponsored by the Kittay
Scientific Foundation, New York, N.Y., March 24-26, 1974).

Interestingly, the conditioning in these animals, made possible by treatment with
amphetamines, persisted after the amphetamines were discontinued. Similarly, animals with a long history of vicious behavior (presumably based on genetic strain and
poor handling by their masters) became gentle very quickly after dosage with amphetamines. Some animals were petted and otherwise treated psychosocially while
receiving amphetamines for six weeks. At the end of this time, amphetamines were
withdrawn and the animals remained "well behaved and lovable" for two years.

The first four of these outcomes are commonly referred to as cures, while the remainder may be viewed at best as treatments of the outward manifestations of the illness.

The highest form of cure is that which treats the illness and prevents its recurrence forever. Such cures are achieved only rarely, as in the case of certain infectious diseases. Thus, immunization techniques purposely induce a minor illness, which results in the generation of sufficient antibodies to protect the host organism for long periods of time or forever—for example, polio, diphtheria, tetanus, pertussis or smallpox.

Slightly lower in the hierarchy is the cure achieved with antibiotics, which eliminate the offending organism; or with vitamins, which make up the deficiency as long as they are taken regularly in the diet.

Still other cures leave residual illness or partial incapacitation, as in the cardiac or renal lesions which may remain following the treatment of streptococcal infections. Often these lesions may persist even though the cause is eliminated.

Surgeons cure by excision: The price of the cure for peptic ulcer may be a partial stomach; for carcinoma of the breast, a mastectomy.

In most of modern medicine, physicians treat rather than cure. Chronic illnesses, frequently of multiple etiology, like hypertension, arthritis, diabetes and the degenerative diseases, are treated for relief of symptoms and to slow or block progression of the illness.

In some illnesses like the common cold, treatment is aimed at relief of symptoms and avoidance of complications while the illness runs its course and spontaneously remits. Treatment goals of this type are quite respectable in medicine, although cures are not achieved. Even the palliative treatments of incurable illnesses which lead to death are considered to be highly desirable forms of treatment while more effective treatments are sought.

There is increasingly greater agreement in psychiatry that the schizophrenias, depression, and perhaps even the neuroses and character disorders, have a multiple etiology; and that for the individual case the quantitative proportions of the constitutional, psychogenic, and immediate causes of the illness are impossible to define. It is therefore somewhat strange that we persistently seek Level 1 cures. In fact, it is doubtful that even with the best treatments now available we are able to treat any form of mental illness so that no scars remain and there is a certainty of no recurrence. More often, we treat, as other physicians do, to remove or minimize symptoms and to rehabilitate socially.

If we relinquish the goal of Level 1 cures as impracticable for the public at large and perhaps even impossible except for those who are not very ill and who are able to afford the time and expense required for prolonged intensive psychotherapy, we must be willing to accept empirical treatments. In this sense the psychopharmacologically minded physician follows in the tradition of most other physicians, who are satisfied with empirical treatments that are effective though perhaps not directly related to the etiology, while they seek more fundamental types of etiologically related treatment through research.

## Study of drug effects needed

Many clinical psychopharmacologists are relatively unconcerned about the psychodynamics of the patient to whom they give drugs. Their primary concern is usually the relief of target symptoms and the social rehabilitation of the patient. To this end, they give minor tranquilizers or sedatives for the relief of neurotic symptoms such as anxiety or insomnia, while simultaneously offering psychotherapy which is more often supportive or directive than intensive. Interestingly, there is an inverse relationship between the frequency of drug use and the nature of the psychotherapy. Intensive or psychoanalytic therapy is associated with a lesser use of drugs than is supportive therapy. An increasing number of clinicians are now using psychotropic agents in combination with group therapy.[5,6]

In the treatment of depression, appropriate antidepressant medication combined with supportive psychotherapy is widely used. The value of these medications has been clearly demonstrated in endogenous depression; it is less certain in reactive depression. The utility of psychotherapy in endogenous depression is uncertain, but it seems clear that the antidepressants facilitate the process of psychotherapy, if only by making the patient more responsive to all aspects of his environment as the depression lifts. In the treatment of acute schizophrenia, the weight of current evidence clearly shows the superiority of drugs over formal psychotherapy during hospitalization,[7] although some therapists still claim better results when drugs are omitted.[8]

Clinical psychopharmacologists do not deny the influence of personality, milieu, social and interpersonal variables in the outcome of drug therapy, but in comparsion to psychodynamically oriented psychiatrists, they tend to minimize the importance of these variables. Thus, Hamilton[9] points out that, with potent drugs in appropriate doses, nonspecific effects diminish: One need not run the usual double-blind placebo controls with vitamin $B_{12}$ in the treatment of pernicious anemia. Equally, one must not be overly influenced by idiosyncratic responses even to simple drugs like alcohol, which may make a given individual euphoric, belligerent or sleepy, depending upon social or other nonspecific factors. But alcohol in appropriate doses makes everyone drunk and uncoordinated, and frequently this constant is more relevant than the other behavioral responses elicited. It is also interesting to note, as Cole *et al*[10] have shown, that in the treatment of schizophrenia nonspecific drug effects are less powerful than specific effects, and that primary symptoms are affected more powerfully than secondary ones. As Hamilton[9] puts it, "Non-specific effects are important for small treatments and small illnesses." With more serious illnesses and more potent treatments, nonspecfic effects become less important.

A second factor contributing toward the failure to integrate psychopharmacology and psychotherapy successfully may lie in the nature of our training programs. Grinker[11] has commented on the degree to which psychodynamics and psychoanalytic concepts are emphasized. This tends to lead to the consideration of psychopharmacology as a second-rate form of treatment to be viewed with some disdain. May,[12] who has addressed himself at length to the problem of psychotherapy and the ataractic drugs, has reviewed several statements by Freud indicating a flexible, tolerant and hopeful attitude toward chemical therapies. But this attitude has rarely been maintained by those who followed him.

A third factor may lie in the nature of the approach in thinking required for comfort with both types of therapy. Psychodynamic theory and its application to practice is subtle, complex, and both intellectually and emotionally seductive to the types of persons who elect the practice of psychiatry as a career. Compared to the richness of this discipline, current teaching of empirical psychopharmacotherapeutics is somewhat pallid.[13] In part this is due to the teaching, which is primarily symptom oriented, rather than syndrome or disease oriented. This emphasis renders it narrowly pragmatic, which tends to preclude the development of a more global and holistic attitude toward the interrelationships between psychodynamics and neurobiology in general, and between psychopathology and psychopharmacological therapeutics in particular. Similar situations are encountered in the teaching of any type of therapeutics throughout medical school. Thus, the teaching of clinical pharmacology has become the province of clinical departments, where it is integrated with concepts of the pathogenesis and specific treatment of disease.

Basic science departments of pharmacology, on the other hand, teach a type of biochemistry and physiology in which drugs are treated as variables that affect normal and pathological metabolic processes according to a predominantly mechanistic and reductionist causal paradigm.

Much of the fundamental research that attempts to relate the action of a drug upon chemical processes within and among neurons to the physiological processes which they subserve and to the behavioral consequences which they generate is both exciting and complex. Although a one-to-one concordance between drugs and discrete chemical processes can be expected, the degree of concordance diminishes as the systems become more complex. The many physical, biochemical and behavioral factors which may influence the response to a drug have been summarized by Irwin[14] (see Table 1 for his summary).

**TABLE 1**

**Factors influencing the response to drugs**

| Physical-Biochemical Factors | Behavioral Factors |
| --- | --- |
| Dosage | Drive state or motivation |
| Route of administration | Affective or mood state |
| Tissue affinity | Level of behavioral activity |
| Tissue responsiveness | Level of sensory input |
| Detoxification rate | Placebo effect |
| Weight, body surface area | Meaning associated with drug |
| Abnormal biochemistry | Defense mechanism interference |
| Tolerance development | Stability of behavior |
| Sex | Complexity of behavior |
| Age | Side effects of drug |

SOURCE: S. Irwin. "Factors Influencing Sensitivity to Stimulant and Depressant Drugs Affecting (a) Loco-motor and (b) Conditioned Avoidance Behavior in Animals," in THE DYNAMICS OF PSYCHIATRIC DRUG THERAPY, G. J. Sarwer-Foner, Ed. (Springfield, Ill.: Charles C Thomas, 1960).

In most cases, our appreciation of the complexity and intellectual challenge of the problem is achieved by personal research efforts involving the anatomy, neurophysiology and biochemistry of the brain and its relationship to behavior, but such research rarely enters into the training experience of the resident. In general, then, the resident learns little more than he gains from the drug literature—that is, the choice of a variety of drugs for specific symptoms, and their doses and side effects. Integrating the drug-relevant material with a detailed grasp of syndromes and illnesses is rarely attempted.

## Developing an integrated theory of drug therapy

In the twenty years since the introduction of psychotropic drugs to American psychiatry, therapeutic practices have changed greatly. The psychotropic drugs have influenced practice far more than they have changed psychiatric theory, but the latter is also changing, thanks to advances in the neurobiological sciences. Still, there remain a number of unresolved problems and conflicts on the theoretical level. The heated debates over the use of drug therapy seem to have subsided, and clinical practice has rapidly accommodated to increasing use of drug therapy. Drug treatments are now prescribed widely, with and without psychotherapy.

These trends with respect to drug therapy may constitute another example of Kuhn's theory of the history of changing scientific ideas. Kuhn[15] proposes that most scientific revolutions are not accomplished by changing the views of a particular group of adherents; rather, a younger generation of scientists and professionals accepts the newer point of view and the older ideas gradually fade because of the death or attrition of their proponents. This may well be the reason for the fading of initial resistance to drug therapy in psychiatric practice. From one point of view, however, it is unfortunate—a number of important theoretical issues generated by the conflict remain unresolved. In particular, the theoretical basis for combined therapy and the nature of interactions between drugs and psychotherapy still remain unclear.

These issues have important implications for the mental health care and delivery system now under scrutiny and criticism in the United States and in other nations. It would obviously be wasteful to combine drugs and psychotherapy if one form of treatment may achieve as much as the combination. Here, as in the health services in general, we need to study not only the relative efficacy of treatments, but also their relative costs. In this respect, the research of Philip May[7] on the psychotherapy and drug therapy of schizophrenia is significant. May has calculated the relative costs and the cost-benefit ratios of various forms of treatment, and has indicated that drug therapy alone, at least during the acute hospitalization phase, has clinical and economic advantages. However, we still need to determine whether these initial advantages have definite long-term value during the rehabilitation and social adjustment phases of posthospital treatment; and particularly whether there is a real place for psychotherapy in the treatment of the discharged patient. For example, it might well be that even if not directly efficacious in itself, supportive psychotherapy has definite indirect effects in successful aftercare, if only by fostering patient compliance with the prescribed chemotherapeutic regimen.

Finally, the lack of an existing comprehensive theory integrating the two ideological approaches is not the only issue. Also and perhaps of primary importance, there is no adequate body of systematic research data concerning the comparative efficacies of various treatments separately and in combination. It is quite possible that we might not be able to develop an integrated theory for some years, but we could at least achieve a broader basis of pragmatic research which would enable us to function more effectively in clinical therapeutics. It is clearly beyond the capacity and scope of this committee to offer a comprehensive theory for mental illness that would account for both biological and psychological determinants. Nor can we precisely specify the proportions of the fashion in which pharmacotherapy and psychotherapy should be used in combination. It is instead our intention to encourage systematic research that will contribute toward a sound and integrated rationale for the various approaches to the treatment of patients, and to illustrate some research designs aimed at achieving such integration.

The problems alluded to in this introduction will therefore be elaborated in what follows by a consideration of the impact on theory and practice of controlled evaluative studies of pharmacotherapy and psychotherapy, alone and in combination, in the treatment of neuroses, depression, and schizophrenia. A consideration of drugs in combination with behavior therapy and with psychoanalysis will also be offered. Finally, some of the practical and methodological problems of research strategy and design will be discussed, which may help to illuminate and resolve some of these problems.

## References

1. J. Levine. Findings quoted in editorial report of frequency of psychotropic drug use, *F.D.C. Reports* 31, 29 (1969): 7.
2. D.I. Manheimer, G.D. Mellinger & M.B. Balter. Psychotherapeutic Drugs: Use Among Adults in California, *California Medicine* 109 (1968): 445.
3. R.M. Whitman. Drugs, Dreams and Experimental Subject, *Canadian Psychiatric Association Journal* 8 (1963): 395.
4. W.T. McKinney, Jr., L.D. Young, S.J. Suomi & J.M. Davis. Chlorpromazine Treatment of Disturbed Monkeys, *Archives of General Psychiatry* 29 (1973): 490.
5. R.C. Cowden & R.C. Finney. Chlorpromazine: Alone and as an Adjunct to Group Therapy in the Treatment of Psychiatric Patients, *American Journal of Psychiatry* 112 (1956): 898.
6. J. Janecek & A. Mandel. The Combined Use of Group and Pharmacotherapy by Collaborative Therapists, *Comprehensive Psychiatry* 6 (1965): 35.

7. P.R.A. May. TREATMENT OF SCHIZOPHRENIA (New York: Science House, 1968).

8. A. Arieti. An Overview of Schizophrenia from a Predominantly Psychological Approach, *American Journal of Psychiatry* 131 (1974): 241.

9. M. Hamilton. "Discussion of the Meeting," in NONSPECIFIC FACTORS IN DRUG THERAPY, K. Rickels, Ed. (Springfield, Ill.: Charles C Thomas, 1968).

10. J. Cole, R. Bonato & S.C. Goldberg. "Nonspecific Factors in Drug Therapy of Schizophrenic Patients," in NONSPECIFIC FACTORS IN DRUG THERAPY, K. Rickels, Ed. (Springfield, Ill.: Charles C Thomas, 1968).

11. R.R. Grinker. A Struggle for Eclecticism, *American Journal of Psychiatry* 121 (1964): 451.

12. P. R. A. May. "Psychotherapy and Ataraxic Drugs," in HANDBOOK OF PSYCHOTHERAPY AND BEHAVIOR CHANGE: AN EMPIRICAL ANALYSIS, A. E. Bergin & S. L. Garfield, Eds. (New York: John Wiley & Sons, 1971).

13. G. L. Klerman. The Teaching of Psychopharmacology in the Psychiatric Residency, *Comprehensive Psychiatry* 6 (1965): 255.

14. S. Irwin. "Factors Influencing Sensitivity to Stimulant and Depressant Drugs Affecting (a) Locomotor and (b) Conditioned Avoidance Behavior in Animals," in THE DYNAMICS OF PSYCHIATRIC DRUG THERAPY, G. J. Sarwer-Foner, Ed. (Springfield, Ill.: Charles C Thomas, 1960).

15. T. S. Kuhn. THE STRUCTURE OF SCIENTIFIC REVOLUTION (Chicago, Ill.: University of Chicago Press, 1962).

# 2

## TREATMENT OF THE NEUROSES AND NONPSYCHOTIC PERSONALITY DISORDERS

### I. NONSPECIFIC FACTORS AND GENERAL METHODOLOGICAL CONSIDERATIONS

An evaluation of the recent studies on the combined treatment of the neuroses is in order. This would also serve to illustrate the principal methodological problems involved in combined drug therapy-psychotherapy research, which will be covered in further detail in Chapter 8.

There is considerable empirical information concerning the pharmacotherapy of the nonpsychotic personality disorders. These data have not as yet been convincingly related to the common belief that the psychoneuroses, character disorders, and impulse disorders are principally caused by adverse experiential factors of a familial, social or cultural type which have led to neurotic conflicts, to social incompetence or deviancy, or to faulty or inefficient habits. From this belief it follows that modification of these disorders involves reeducation, retraining, and rehabilitation—or psychotherapy in its most general sense. Since the evaluation of the effectiveness of psychotherapy in its many forms is itself a formidable problem, small wonder that the use of psychoactive drugs as agents to effect personality change presents formidable problems in evaluative research.

The principal methodological problems involved in the design and execution of studies in combined drug therapy-psychotherapy research are discussed in detail in Chapter 8. Here, the primary consideration is the evaluation of the results of some recent experimental work in the study of the combined treatment of the neuroses. However, certain qualitative and relatively nonspecific factors that may influence the observed pharmacological profile of psychoactive drugs or that may be relevant to the technique and outcome of psychotherapy must be given due attention.

## 1. Changes over time in untreated psychiatric patients

There is evidence that symptomatic improvement occurs spontaneously in a relatively high proportion of untreated psychiatric patients. Eysenck's reviews of the literature[1-3] led him to raise the question whether psychotherapy does any better than no such therapy or even the mere passage of time. Scholarly and erudite rebuttals in the literature to Eysenck's arguments by Luborsky,[4] Rosenzweig,[5] and 14 other prominent scholars[3] have not entirely reassured the scientific community that psychotherapy is a definite causal agent in changing personality and behavior disorders.

One of the major problems in the assessment of the "natural history" of emotional illness has been the difficulty of obtaining patients who are in fact untreated. Many patients who consult a psychiatrist have already received some form of interpersonal assistance or guidance under medical or nonmedical auspices, given by a nonpsychiatric physician, a psychologist, a sociologist, a social worker, a clergyman or a nonprofessional counselor. Nonspecific factors in treatment (i.e., the interest of one human being in the problems of another, the simple act of communication between two or more individuals, the expression of sympathy and encouragement by the counselor or therapist) may be a major determinant in producing at least transient alleviation of symptoms. Therefore, various compromises have to be made about what constitutes a truly "untreated" patient. What are some of the findings coming from such studies?

**a—Psychoneurotic patients receiving little treatment or nonspecific treatment:** Denker[6] followed up treatment by general prac-

titioners of 500 consecutive disability claims for neurosis from
the files of an insurance company. He found that after 2
years, 72% of the patients, and after 5 years, 90%, were
"able to return to work and carry on well in both their
economic and social adjustments." Although there is the possibility here of compensation neurosis rather than true spontaneous remission, these data are nonetheless highly
suggestive.[7]

Ernst,[8] using purely symptomatic criteria, found an improvement rate among mixed psychoneurotic patients of 77%
(N = 120) with an average follow-up of 24 years.

Malan et al[9] attempted to evaluate the symptomatic improvement of untreated neurotic patients from a psychodynamic point of view. In a 2- to 8-year follow-up study of 45
untreated patients at the Tavistock Clinic, 51% were found to
be symptomatically "improved" and 20% symptomatically
"recovered." Out of the "improved" group, 29% were judged
still psychodynamically "suspect"—that is, still showed evidence of a heightened propensity to neurotic symptom formation although their initial symptoms were relatively qui-
escent. By the same psychodynamic criterion, in the
"recovered" group 18% showed persisting evidence of
neurosis. In summary, of these 45 untreated patients, only
22% were found to be "improved" from the psychodynamic
point of view (vs. 51% from the symptomatic viewpoint), and
only 2% (1 patient) were judged "recovered" (vs. 20% "recovered" from the symptomatic viewpoint).

Muller[10] found a symptomatic improvement rate of 49% (N
= 57) with a follow-up of 5 years and for more than half the
patients over 20 years. His criteria for "improved" were: socially adapted, able to work, relatively good human relations,
obsessional symptoms still present but clearly much milder.

Saslow and Peters[11] followed up, 1 to 7 years after initial
contact, 87 out of 100 consecutive patients, diagnosed as having a behavior disorder, who had had not more than two

interviews. Criteria of change were those of Miles *et al.*[12] Thirty-seven percent were evaluated as "apparently recovered" to "improved."

Wallace and Whyte[13] followed up 49 out of 76 patients who had been on a waiting list for psychotherapy for 3 to 7 years but had not received treatment. Sixty-five percent were found to be "recovered" or "improved." The criteria for "recovered" were: symptom-free, fully employed, and no loss of socioeconomic status. The criteria for "improved" were: patient troubled only by residual symptoms, fully employed, and no loss in socioeconomic status.

**b—Untreated controls compared with treated patients, or less specifically treated patients compared with more specifically treated patients:** Barron and Leary[14] found no significant difference between treated and waiting-list psychoneurotic patients 7-8 months after initial contact, using M.M.P.I. criteria as change measures.

Brill[15] found no significant differences after 2 years among M.M.P.I. criteria for a group of women patients with chronic character disorders, using psychotherapy (administered by medical students), as compared to a group of similar women who were put on a waiting list but never received treatment.

Cremerius[16] found that psychosomatic patients were significantly better symptomatically 8-10 years after receiving analytically oriented psychotherapy than a group of similar patients after receiving less "specific" treatment.

Endicott and Endicott[17] found no significant differences between patients receiving psychotherapy and patients who were waiting list controls in the scores of various psychological tests, the M.M.P.I., and clinical rating scales, 6 months after therapy.

Rogers and Dymond[18] found significantly greater improvement in such criteria as self-ideal correlation, clinical evaluation, and certain T.A.T. dimensions 2 months after psychotherapy, as compared to the status of waiting list controls.

Shlien *et al*[19] reported significantly greater improvement in self-ideal correlation 3 months after psychotherapy, as compared to the same correlation in waiting list controls.

Stone *et al*[20] reported significantly greater improvement in the criterion of social ineffectiveness after 6 months (but not after 5 years) among a group of patients receiving psychotherapy, as compared to a group receiving "minimal contact therapy" (not more than 30 minutes once a fortnight). No treatment-related differences were noted in improvement of symptomatic discomfort.

## 2. Effects of placebos

Careful psychopharmacological research almost always involves the use of placebo-drug comparisons. This type of control is useful in assessing the extent to which the active drug is a causal agent in symptomatic or personality changes. Comparison of treatment outcomes using psychotherapy in combination with active drug or placebo is useful in pinning down causal relationships, although such a research design requires larger numbers of patients than simpler designs.

To consider what effect the introduction of a placebo into a psychopharmacological study might have on study results, it would be helpful to look briefly at the psychological reactions which can be elicited by placebos. Several reviews of the effects of placebo[21-27] have clearly indicated its power in relation to symptomatic change. Rickels[28] reports that even the dose level of placebo can be instrumental in inducing a placebo effect or in reversing a placebo-drug difference: In this study, chlordiazepoxide or barbiturate dosage was found to be associated with a significant alleviation of symptoms, as compared to the effect of 4 placebo capsules per day but not as compared to 8 placebo capsules daily.

Evidence has been provided that the placebo effect is not necessarily associated with suggestibility or with hypnotizability. The effect is often inconstant for the individual and may be more likely to occur under special circumstances, such as under the stress of pain after surgery, when a placebo is used as a "pain killer."[23] Moreover, the placebo effect is often quite short-lived in comparison to the effect of a pharmacologically active medicament. Nonetheless, the placebo effect is clearly not to be written off as spurious, "merely imaginary," or somehow "less real" than the effect of an active drug, as it sometimes is by "tough-minded" clinicians and researchers. The optimism and confidence engendered by the utilization of any treatment modality the patient really believes will help him are not necessarily the product of magical thinking, but rather can be a crucial factor in altering the patient's mental set and thus his further psychotherapeutic progress. In this way, a positive placebo effect may actually augment the therapeutic efficacy even of pharmacologically active agents. The discussion which follows is relevant to this important issue of securing and maintaining a positive, constructive attitude on the part of the patient.

## 3. Effect of psychotherapeutic goal(s)

The goals of the psychotherapies differ considerably. A psychotherapeutic program aimed at increasing the affect experienced by an obsessive-compulsive patient probably will require an adjunctive drug different from that required by a psychotherapeutic program aimed at decreasing the current affective level or arousal capacity of the individual. Hence, the psychotherapist must carefully consider his goals, short-term and long, before prescribing a drug to accompany his psychotherapy.

More subtly, when the therapeutic goal involves a hoped-for change in a complex character trait, probably the psychotherapist should not only provide a rational explanation to his patient for prescribing a medicament, but he should also distinguish the short-term versus the long-term aspects of the drug component of his therapeutic regimen.

At present it would be foolhardy to attempt to state in a formula what the rationale of drug administration should be in the treatment of nonpsychotic patients, for this field of therapeutics is too new to insist on such precision. There is considerable room for careful experimentation in this area—not haphazard, unplanned clinical investigation, but rather psychoactive drug studies with sound research design and controls, explicit formulations, and all the other features of a well-planned research project.

Some current uses of psychoactive drugs in combination with psychoactive treatment of nonpsychotic personality disorders may be noted here:

1. To inhibit, alleviate or suppress symptoms, such as anxiety, hostility or panic attacks.
2. To combat insomnia.
3. To stimulate energy, psychomotor activity, creativity.
4. To induce and maintain rapport with the psychotherapist.
5. To reduce irrational fear (as in phobia) as a step in a program of psychotherapy so that the patient will try to carry out the neurotically feared activity. There is no evidence that at appropriate dosages psychoactive drugs which inhibit anxiety—that is, irrational fear—also decrease the intensity of realistic fear.
6. To decrease irrational affects moderately to a level where the patient's observing ego, his more rational self, can function sufficiently well to gain understanding of his conflicts through psychotherapy.
7. To allay the patient's inertia or paralyzing depressive mood so that he can function domestically and vocationally, and can collaborate effectively with the psychotherapist.
8. To reinforce suggestions of the psychotherapist.
9. To suppress periodic psychotic thinking or behavior.
10. To induce altered states of consciousness, as in psychedelic drug treatment.

## 4. Effect of therapist's personality

The effects of the psychotherapist's personality and his attitude toward the patient on the outcome of treatment have been studied assiduously for many years by psychoanalysts,[29] and more recently by "nondirective" or "client-centered" therapists.[7,30-33] These studies indicate that the attitude or personality of the therapist may often profoundly influence both the immediate and the subsequent course of psychotherapy. Some psychotherapists seem to achieve patient improvement regularly and some to achieve patient deterioration.[31,33-41] Even in brief 5-minute interviews where standardized instructions for eliciting speech from the subject are read and where the interviewer is silent during this time, maintaining an unreactive facial expression, a content analysis of the subject's verbal behavior has shown significantly greater anxiety and hostility regularly expressed with some interviewers as compared to others.[42,43]

It is highly likely that with the usual therapeutic doses of the typical drugs used in the treatment of the nonpsychotic personality disorders, the personality and attitude of the therapist also influence the drug effect noted in pharmacotherapy. Several investigators studying the relative effectiveness of different psychoactive drugs with outpatients, as administered by different physicians, where no formalized psychotherapy was carried out, have reported different results associated with different physicians.[28,44,45]

## 5. Effect of patient's personality

Some effects of the patient's personality on recovery are well known to every practicing clinician. A high percentage of patients with acute anxiety or neurotic depression but with otherwise well-adjusted personality make-up recover readily with almost any form of therapy (see previous discussion of change in "untreated" psychoneurotic patients). Given enough time, one-half to two-thirds experience alleviation of their symptoms with the passage of time alone, although underlying psychodynamic changes may fail to occur.[9]

An indication of the influence of personality make-up on change over time in psychoneurotic patients receiving little or no therapy of any kind is suggested by the study of Endicott and Endicott.[17] They studied certain demographic and personality characteristics of 40 outpatients who improved after being kept on a waiting list without formal psychiatric treatment for approximately 6 months. Twelve clinical rating scales were used. The "improved" group showed lower initial (pre-wait) ratings on the Depression and Hostility scales and significantly higher initial ratings on scales of Self-Esteem, Adaptation to Reality Testing, Thought Processes, Defenses, Ego Strength, and Mental Health. Furthermore, the "improved" group had significantly more education than the "unimproved" group. Also, the "improved" group showed lower scores on the Pa and F scales of the M.M.P.I., higher scores on the Rorschach Prognostic Scale, and larger mean numbers of FC and Rorschach responses than the "unimproved" group.

Gottschalk et al[46] have pursued the question of what personality traits typify those acutely upset psychiatric patients who improve the most, primarily with brief (six treatment sessions or fewer) psychoanalytically oriented psychotherapy and sparing use of psychoactive drugs. Good responders were found to have the following characteristics: (a) a facility and positive interest in interpersonal object relationships (high score on the Gottschalk Human Relations Verbal Behavior Scale); (b) relatively little thinking disorder or social alienation (low social alienation-personal disorganization score on the Gottschalk-Gleser Verbal Behavior Scale); (c) acutely disabling psychological symptoms (high scores on the Gottschalk Psychiatric Morbidity Scale and the Gottschalk-Gleser Anxiety and Hostility Inward Scales); and (d) membership in the lower socioeconomic classes (social classes IV and V of the Hollingshead-Redlich Scale). The importance of the patient's personality in his response to psychotherapy has been documented by many other investigators as well.[39,40,47-49]

A number of authors have reported studies on the influence of the patient's personality on the effects of psychoactive drugs.[28,35,50,51] McNair *et al*,[52] for example, showed that patients scoring low on the Bass Social Acquiescence Scale responded better to a minor tranquilizer than to placebo, whereas high-scoring patients responded equally as well to placebo as to the drug.

Rickels *et al*[53] showed that depressed patients in a medical clinic responded better to meprobamate-benactyzine than to imipramine, whereas depressed patients in a psychiatric clinic responded about the same to the two medications. The medical clinic patients were of lower socioeconomic class, were more somatically focused and more drug-oriented, and regarded the physician as a powerful authority figure.

Rickels,[28] summarizing several years' study of nonspecific factors in drug response, makes the point that in many respects patients who respond well to an active drug resemble those who are commonly believed to be suitable only for psychotherapy.

Grosser[54] found that depressed patients of the lower and upper social classes did not respond as well to drugs as did middle-class patients. Wittenborn[55] described an excessively dependent, self-critical, premorbid personality in depressed patients as a negative prognostic sign for response to imipramine, but not to iproniazid. He has also provided a good review of patient characteristics which aid in the prediction of response to antidepressant medication.[56]

## 6. Effect of patient's mental set

Apart from the personality of the therapist or the patient, the effect of treatment also depends on the mental set or expectations of the patient about the effects of treatment. This has been amply documented among patients in psychotherapy by such workers as Frank[57] and Goldstein.[58] Both Friedman[59] and Uhlenhuth and Duncan,[40] for example, found that patients who initially expected greater improvement did improve more in psychotherapy than those without such expectations.

Likewise, the effect of a drug can be influenced by the patient's expectations about it.[60] In an experimental double-blind placebo study, Gottschalk et al[61] noted that telling subjects they could expect to feel "more peppy and energetic" after ingesting a pill resulted in significant increases in achievement strivings (as measured by a verbal content analysis procedure), whether or not the subject received a placebo, secobarbital (100 mg.), or dextroamphetamine (10 mg.). Less surprisingly, the administration of dextroamphetamine led to significantly higher achievement-striving scores (based on the same content analysis scale) than either of the other psychoactive agents and regardless of the induced mental set. The effects of the dextroamphetamine and the induced mental set were additive and resulted in greater achievement-striving scores when the drug and the mental set were given together. These findings, however, did not generalize to other psychological states, such as provoking greater or less anxiety or hostility with several combinations of these drugs and mental sets.

Fisher et al[62] and Uhlenhuth et al[45] found that under some circumstances the effect of a mild tranquilizer was more marked when it was described to patients as a specific remedy than when it was described as an experimental drug for evaluation.

Finally, it is worth noting that quantitative studies suggest a variety of other factors as influencing response to treatment. Among these are the general treatment milieu[63] and the intercurrent life event.[64]

The clinician must be fully aware of these considerations when determining his treatment strategy for a given patient or a clinically similar group of patients. Ideally, however, sound clinical practice should be based upon and substantiated by systematic research designed to assess various treatment modalities alone and in combination. Although the value of pharmacotherapy in the treatment of the neuroses has been substantiated by controlled studies to a lesser extent than it has in other areas of psychiatric practice (e.g., the proven efficacy of the phenothiazines in the schizophrenias), it is clear that there is great potential in the appropriate use of psychoactive agents for the treatment of the nonpsychotic personality disorders. Therefore, a review of some of the literature reporting recent studies in combined psychotherapy and pharmacotherapy in this area may be useful.

## II.  CONTROLLED CLINICAL TRIALS EVALUATING DRUG-PSYCHOTHERAPY INTERACTION

Carefully controlled studies employing an adequate experimental design and a sufficient number of matched patients are difficult to perform (see Chapter 8). Consequently, there are singularly few studies in the psychiatric literature involving combined pharmacotherapy and psychotherapy which fully satisfy rigorous scientific criteria.

Double-blind placebo-controlled drug studies have described a wide variety of modifiable symptoms and signs. Examples include reduction in primary-process thinking (as well as the more typical effect of alleviating target anxiety) by chlordiazepoxide[65]; and increase of achievement strivings induced by dextroamphetamine.[61] Other studies have provided evidence in nonpsychotic individuals of the anxiety- and/or hostility-alleviating effects of many tranquilizers and sedatives—for example, perphenazine,[66] chlordiazepoxide,[67] diazepam,[68,69] lorazepam,[70] and barbiturates.[71] Repeated doses of the energizers among subjects with nonpsychotic personality disorders have been reported to increase anxiety and hostility outward.[72] On the other hand, there are reports indicating that under certain conditions some psychoactive drugs may have no more influence on these affective variables than a placebo.[51,73]

An early double-blind study of combined pharmacotherapy (chronic dosage) and psychotherapy in predominantly psychoneurotic outpatients was reported by Lorr *et al*,[74] in which 180 male veterans participated. They received weekly individual psychotherapy alone, or psychotherapy combined with chlorpromazine (100 mgm. daily), meprobamate (1600 mgm.), phenobarbital (130 mgm.), or placebo. The 50-minute psychotherapeutic hours were conducted mainly by experienced therapists. After 8 weeks, all treatment groups showed about the same decrease in a variety of symptoms. The three groups receiving drugs, however, showed some increase in hostility. All medications were then discontinued, although patients continued to come for psychotherapy. After 4 more weeks, hostility had dropped to the pretreatment level and patients who had taken phenobarbital showed somewhat less symptomatic improvement than the rest. On the whole, however, no important differences were noted among treatment groups and no significant changes from the 8-week evaluation period.

In a sequel to this study, Lorr *et al*[75] investigated the early effects of a minor tranquilizer, chlordiazepoxide, at a flexible dosage, under conditions closely resembling their previous study. Those tested were divided into six treatment groups: (1) chlordiazepoxide with psychotherapy, (2) chlordiazepoxide without psychotherapy, (3) placebo with psychotherapy, (4) placebo without psychotherapy, (5) psychotherapy alone, and (6) no treatment. After 1 week, the patients' reports showed the drug to be more effective than placebo and that both capsules were more effective than no capsules. After 4 weeks, however, the patients' reports showed only that capsules were more effective than no capsules. No longer were there differences between drug and placebo, nor were there differences between psychotherapy and no psychotherapy. Interactions between treatments were observed only on a single criterion measure—the level of somatic discomfort: Chlordiazepoxide was superior to placebo for patients who received psychotherapy, whereas all capsules were superior to no capsules for patients who did not receive psychotherapy.

According to the therapists' reports, after 4 weeks chlordiazepoxide was judged more effective than placebo; capsules were more effective than no capsules; and especially significant was the therapists' judgment that patients who received chlordiazepoxide showed greater rapport in interviews. The medication was not found to impede the interview relationship with any patient and it facilitated psychotherapy for about one-third of patients.

Roth *et al*[76] followed the patients from the preceding study over a further 6 months of psychotherapy, combined with medication at the therapist's discretion. Measures of major outcome were therapists' ratings of symptom relief, gain in competence, personality gain, and global success, each on a 5-point scale. Ratings of these criteria showed that patients who had started on psychotherapy improved most. There was also some indication of interaction between the initial psychotherapy and conditions of medication: Patients who had started on psychotherapy (alone, with placebo, or with chlordiazepoxide) or on chlordiazepoxide alone tended to progress equally well, whereas patients who had started on placebo alone or on no treatment tended to progress relatively less well.

These three related studies suggest that a minor tranquilizer added to psychotherapy by experienced therapists accelerates symptomatic improvement and facilitates the psychotherapeutic exchange. The second study implies that the early effects of the combined treatments may be additive. Both the first and the third studies suggest that, over longer periods, two effective treatments combined produce about the same benefit as each treatment alone. In none of these studies, however, is the picture of interaction between treatments clear and incontestable. The inconclusiveness of these three studies is in part attributable to deficiencies in design. Male veterans represent a unique population.

Lorr and Roth repeatedly referred to the use of experienced psychotherapists and psychiatrists, but the nature of their experience is never fully defined. May emphasizes that the whole area of experience is a very shady one. How does one equate the experience of a psychologist and a psychiatrist? Is it measurable in years of patient care, or by the number of psychiatric cases previously treated? May also emphasizes that skill and experience in drug usage may be every bit as important as skill and experience in psychotherapy. Altogether we tend to make the naïve assumption that skill in pharmacotherapy can be derived from the package insert while years of training are required for experience in psychotherapy.

Once-a-week psychotherapy may be far from the optimum, and the nature of the psychotherapy is not fully explicated. In the first study the role of psychotherapy is difficult to evaluate, because this study furnishes no direct information about the effectiveness of the psychotherapy employed. The same comment applies to the long-term psychotherapy offered in the third study. In this study, furthermore, the effects of long-term pharmacotherapy upon outcome are not analyzed, even though significant differences in regard to drug prescription among treatment groups are noted.

A serious shortcoming of these studies is the small fraction of entering patients who actually figured in the final analyses. Results were based on 58% of initial sample in the first study and on 48% of initial sample in the second study. In the second study, moreover, the rate of dropout was higher for patients who received psychotherapy than for those who did not. More striking treatment differences and interaction patterns may have been obscured by the attrition of both the most-improved and the least-improved patients.[77] Finally, the unavoidable possibility of bias in some of the therapists' ratings must be acknowledged.

Rickels *et al*[78] studied the effects of meprobamate, 1600 mgm. daily, or placebo, each combined with psychotherapy provided by 5 experienced private psychiatrists in their offices. A total of 114 patients participated. Medications were assigned at random and under double-blind conditions. Psychotherapeutic interviews lasting from less than 30 minutes to about 45 minutes took place once weekly. Assessments were made every 2 weeks over the total study period of 6 weeks. After 2 weeks, the patients' global ratings and the physicians' global ratings and individual symptom ratings showed no drug-placebo differences. After 4 and 6 weeks, however, most of these ratings showed that meprobamate was more effective than placebo.

In this study, then, a minor tranquilizer produced benefit when combined with psychotherapy. This additional benefit increased as treatment progressed. The authors pointed out but did not really attempt to reconcile the contradictions between their results and those of Lorr's group. The descriptions of the studies, however, suggest gross differences in the psychotherapy offered by the two groups of investigators. The amount of psychotherapeutic contact in the Rickels study was (1) more variable and (2) less, on the average than in the Lorr studies. Unfortunately, the data do not indicate duration of the average interview in the Rickels study. Patients may have responded more to medication in this study because the low psychotherapeutic contact was ineffective.[79] It is worth considering the further possibility that patients in this study responded more to medication because these 5 therapists on the average were less effective than Lorr's therapists. These questions cannot be resolved, since the design of the Rickels study did not provide for an estimate of psychotherapeutic effect alone.

Rickels and Cattell[80] further analyzed the results of this study in terms of medication, type of doctor, and the interaction between these two variables. On psychological testing, Group I doctors were authoritarian, extraverted and Betz-Whitehorn type A. Group II doctors were less authoritarian and extraverted and were Betz-Whitehorn type B. Patients treated with placebo by Group I doctors responded less favorably than patients in the other three treatment conditions. Patients in this study were assigned at random to medication, but each doctor selected patients from his own practice. Comparison of patient characteristics between doctor types revealed that the patients of Group I doctors were sicker, older, and less educated; more of them were chronically ill, had been pretreated with drugs, and were more drug oriented than those of Group II doctors—in short, poorer candidates for psychotherapy alone. It was therefore impossible to ascertain whether doctor type or patient characteristics played the crucial role in the interaction with medication effects. Nevertheless, the results do point up more clearly some possible sources of the disagreement with Lorr's group.

Wittenborn[81] analyzed two large bodies of standardized clinical reports on anxious patients who took oxazepam, chlordiazepoxide or placebo. These patients were not subjects of a designed study, but study results are of interest because of the large number of patients involved and the author's imaginative use of statistical controls. His 1963 total sample of 944 patients showed a clearly superior response in the alleviation of anxiety and tension with the tranquilizers as compared to placebo. The 417 patients treated by psychiatrists, however, did not respond differentially to drug and placebo. The psychiatrists' patients and the other medical specialists' patients responded equally well to drug, but the psychiatrists' patients responded much better to placebo than did the other specialists' patients. The results in Wittenborn's 1963 total sample were closely replicated by his 1964 sample. The 352 patients treated by psychiatrists in 1964, however, gave results consistent with the total 1963 sample. The patients treated by psychiatrists in 1963 apparently had less psychotherapy than those treated in 1964. Unfortunately the data were not entirely adequate in this regard.

Chassan[82] has presented an interesting approach to studying the effects in psychoneurotic outpatients of minor tranquilizers combined with psychotherapy. He advocates close study of the individual patient's responses to multiple double-blind, placebo-controlled alternations of medication, by means of frequently repeated patient assessments. He makes the assumption that long-term trend of improvement represents the effect of psychotherapy, so that the effects of the alternating medications can be determined by progressively evaluating the patient's clinical status on the basis of interval observations and then at termination of the study period, correlating these assessments with the on-drug, off-drug periods. He calls this approach "intensive design." With this technique, Bellak and Chassan[65] reported that chlordiazepoxide relieved a variety of symptoms more effectively than placebo in a single patient concurrently participating in psychotherapy.

McLaughlin et al[83] found that the relative effectiveness of diazepam, meprobamate and placebo differed in three different patients. Unfortunately, in this study the authors could not define the source of disagreement in the three results, since the 3 patients, and perhaps their treatment as well, differed in so many respects. Unrecognized carry-over effects from one medication period to the next may have affected the results; or possibly undetected interactions between the medi-

cations and other treatment factors, particularly psychotherapy, may well have been operative.

In their most recent work, Bellak *et al* employed their "intensive design" in a longitudinal study of ego function of a
single case receiving psychoanalytic psychotherapy. In a
double-blind design the patient periodically received or was
taken off diazepam while psychotherapy was continued. The
results showed significant global improvement as well as improvement in specific ego functions which they attributed to
the drug.

Jacobs *et al*[84] used a particularly interesting form of intensive design directed toward revealing at least short-term interactions between medication and psychotherapy. In their
study, 8 patients reported distress during the preceding week
and distress immediately before and after each weekly interview. These patients reported the same relief across the interview when they were taking diazepam and when they were
taking placebo. There was some suggestion, however, that
they experienced greater relief in anticipation of the interview when they were taking placebo than when they were
taking diazepam. As the authors point out, this apparent
interaction may have been related simply to the patient's
overall level of distress during the week before the interview
("law of initial value"), since the patients were more distressed
during placebo weeks than during diazepam weeks. Unfortunately, the analyses necessary to test this very plausible interpretation were not performed.

## FURTHER RESEARCH NEEDED

Although the number of studies is not great and the results
are skimpy and inconclusive, they do provide evidence that
such research is feasible, as well as some tentative working
hypotheses for predicting which psychiatric patients might
improve without formal treatment by some method of

psychotherapy or with some psychoactive drug. It is likely that different predictors will be found for different types and combinations of therapies, but there may well be considerable overlap among the relevant personality strengths and weaknesses of the patient. Certainly for many acute psychiatric disorders, the patient's own self-curative capacities may be of major importance. In any event, we need to be careful about prematurely attributing change which occurs during treatment to any single component of that treatment. Only further extensive and carefully controlled research will provide us with conclusive answers to the pressing questions, What is the optimally effective treatment of the neurotic patient and what is the value of combined treatments?

## References

1. H.J. Eysenck. The Effects of Psychotherapy, An Evaluation, *Journal of Consulting Psychology* 16 (1952): 319.
2. _____. HANDBOOK OF ABNORMAL PSYCHOLOGY (London, England: Isaac Pitman, 1960).
3. _____. The Effects of Psychotherapy (with discussions by 14 prominent psychotherapists), *International Journal of Psychiatry* 1 (1965): 97.
4. L. Luborsky. A Note on Eysenck's Article, "The Effects of Psychotherapy, an Evaluation," *British Journal of Psychology* 45 (1954): 129.
5. S. Rosenzweig. A Transvaluation of Psychotherapy: A Reply to Hans Eysenck, *Journal of Abnormal & Social Psychology* 49 (1954): 298.
6. P.G. Denker. Results of Treatment of Psychoneurosis by the General Practitioner, *New York State Journal of Medicine* 46 (1946): 2164.
7. A.E. Bergin. "An Empirical Analysis of Therapeutic Issues," in COUNSELING AND PSYCHOTHERAPY: AN OVERVIEW, D. Arbuckle, Ed. (New York: McGraw-Hill Press, 1967).
8. K. Ernst. "Die Prognose der Neurosen," in MONOGRAPHIEN AUS

DEM GESAMTGEBIETE DER NEUROLOGIE UND PSYCHIATRIE, Heft 85 (Berlin, Gottingen, Heidelberg: Springer, 1950).

9. D.H. Malan, H.A. Bacal, E.S. Heath, & F.H.G. Balfour. A Study of Psychodynamic Changes in Untreated Neurotic Patients, *British Journal of Psychiatry* 114 (1968): 525.

10. C. Müller. Vorläufige Mitteilung zur langen Katamnese der Zwangskranken, *Nervenarzt* 24 (1953): 112.

11. G. Saslow & A. Peters. A Follow-up Study of "Untreated" Patients with Various Behavior Disorders, *Psychiatric Quarterly* 30 (1956): 283.

12. H. Miles, E. Barrabee & J. Finesinger. Evaluation of Psychotherapy, *Psychosomatic Medicine* 13 (1951): 82.

13. H.E.R. Wallace & M.B.H. Whyte. Natural History of the Psychoneurosis, *British Medical Journal* 1 (1959): 144.

14. F. Barron & T.F. Leary. Changes in Psychoneurotic Patients with and without Psychotherapy. *Journal of Consulting Psychology* 19 (1955): 239.

15. N.Q. Brill, Results of Psychotherapy, *California Medicine* 104 (1966): 249.

16. J. Cremerius. "Die Beurteilung des Behandlungserfolges in der Psychotherapie," in MONOGRAPHIEN AUS DEM GESAMTGEBIETE DER NEUROLOGIE UND PSYCHIATRIE Heft 99 (Gottingen, Heidelberg: Springer 1962).

17. N.A. Endicott & J. Endicott. Improvement in Untreated Psychiatric Patients, *Archives of General Psychiatry* 9 (1963): 575.

18. C.R. Rogers & F. Dymond. PSYCHOTHERAPY AND PERSONALITY CHANGE (Chicago, Ill.: University of Chicago Press, 1954).

19. J.M. Shlien, H.H. Mosak & R. Dreikurs. Effect of Time Limits: A Comparison of Two Psychotherapies, *Counseling Psychology* 9 (1962): 31.

20. A.R. Stone, J.D. Frank, E.H. Nash & S.D. Imbers. An Intensive Five-year Follow-up Study of Treated Psychiatric Outpatients, *Journal of Nervous & Mental Disease* 133 (1961): 410.

21. S. Wolf. Effects of Suggestion and Conditioning on the Action of Chemical Agents in Human Subjects: The Pharmacology of Placebos, *Journal of Clinical Investigation* 29 (1950): 100.

22. H.K. Beecher. The Powerful Placebo, *Journal of the American Medical Association* 159 (1955): 1602.

23. _____. Surgery as Placebo: A Quantitative Study of Bias, *Journal of the American Medical Association* 176 (1961): 1102.

24. R.M. Steinbook, M. Jones & J.D. Ainslie. Suggestibility and the Placebo Response, *Journal of Nervous and Mental Disease* 140 (1965): 87.

25. L.C. Park & L. Covi. Non-blind Placebo Trial: An Exploration of Neurotic Patients' Responses to Placebo When Its Inert Content Is Disclosed, *Archives of General Psychiatry* 12 (1966): 36.

26. D.M. Gelfand, S. Gelfand & M.W. Rardin. Some Personality Factors Associated with Placebo Responsitivity, *Psychological Reports* 17 (1965): 555.

27. B.P. Muller. Personality of Placebo Reactors and Non-reactors, *Diseases of the Nervous System* 26 (1965): 58.

28. K. Rickels. NONSPECIFIC FACTORS IN DRUG THERAPY, (Springfield, Ill.: Charles C Thomas, 1968).

29. D. Orr. Transference and Countertransference: A Historical Survey, *Journal of the American Psychoanalytic Association* 2 (1954): 621.

30. A.E. Bergin. The Effects of Psychotherapy: Negative Results Revisited, *Journal of Counseling Psychology* 10 (1963): 244.

31. _____. Some Implications of Psychotherapy Research for Therapeutic Practice, *International Journal of Psychiatry* 3 (1967): 136.

32. J.M. Shlien & F.M. Zimring. "Research Directives and Methods in Client Centered Therapy," in METHODS OF RESEARCH IN PSYCHOTHERAPY, L.A. Gottschalk & A.H. Auerbach, Eds. (New York: Appleton-Century-Crofts, 1966).

33. C.B. Truax & R.R. Carkhuff. TOWARD EFFECTIVE COUNSELING AND PSYCHOTHERAPY: TRAINING AND PRACTICE. (Chicago, Ill.: Aldine Publishing, 1967).

34. R.D. Cartwright & J.L. Vogel. A Comparison of Changes in Psychoneurotic Patients During Matched Periods of Therapy and No Therapy, *Journal of Consulting Psychology* 24 (1960): 121.

35. R.R. Kogler & N.Q. Brill. TREATMENT OF PSYCHIATRIC OUTPATIENTS (New York: Appleton-Century-Crofts, 1967).

36. M. Lorr & D.M. McNair. "Methods Relating to Evaluation of Therapeutic Outcome," in METHODS OF RESEARCH IN PSYCHOTHERAPY, L.A. Gottschalk & A.H. Auerbach, Eds. (New York: Appleton-Century-Crofts, 1966).

37. D.M. McNair, D.M. Callahan & M. Lorr. Therapist "Type" and Patient Response to Psychotherapy, *Journal of Consulting Psychology* 26 (1962): 425.
38. J.K. Myers & F. Auld. Some Variables Related to Outcome of Psychotherapy, *Journal of Clinical Psychology* 11 (1955): 51.
39. E.H. Nash, R. Hoehn-Saric, C.C. Battle, A.R. Stone, S.D. Imber & J.D. Frank. Systematic Preparation of Patients for Short-term Psychotherapy: II. Relation to Characteristics of Patient, Therapist and the Psychotherapeutic Process, *Journal of Nervous & Mental Disease* 140 (1965): 374.
40. E.H. Uhlenhuth & D.B. Duncan. Subjective Change with Medical Student Therapists: II. Some Determinants of Change in Psychoneurotic Outpatients, *Archives of General Psychiatry* 18 (1968): 532.
41. J.C. Whitehorn & B.J. Betz. A Study of Psychotherapeutic Relationships between Physicians and Schizophrenic Patients, *American Journal of Psychiatry* 111 (1954): 321.
42. L.A. Gottschalk. "Some Problems in the Evaluation of Psychoactive Drugs, with and without Psychotherapy, in the Treatment of Nonpsychotic Personality Disorders," in PSYCHOPHARMACOLOGY: A REVIEW OF PROGRESS, 1957-1967, D.H. Efron, J.O. Cole, J. Levine & J.R. Wittenborn, Eds. PHS Pub. No. 1836 (Washington, D.C.: Govt. Ptg. Ofc., 1968).
43. _____. Some Psychoanalytic Research into the Communication of Meaning Through Language: The Quality and Magnitude of Psychological States, *British Journal of Medical Psychology* 44 (1971): 131-148.
44. M.H. Sheard. The Influence of the Doctor's Attitude on the Patients' Response to Antidepressant Medication, *Journal of Nervous & Mental Disease* 136 (1963): 555.
45. E.H. Uhlenhuth, K. Rickels, S. Fisher, L.C. Park, R.S. Lysman & J. Mock. Drug, Doctor's Verbal Attitude, and Clinic Setting in the Symptomatic Response to Pharmacotherapy, *Psychopharmacologia*, (1966): 392.
46. L.A. Gottschalk, P. Mayerson & A. Gottlieb. The Prediction and Evaluation of Outcome in an Emergency Brief Psychotherapy Clinic, *Journal of Nervous & Mental Disease* 144 (1967): 77.
47. F. Barron. An Ego-strength Scale Which Predicts Response to Psychotherapy, *Journal of Consulting Psychology* 17 (1953): 327.

48. S.D. Imber, E.H. Nash, R. Hoehn-Saric, A.R. Stone & J.D. Frank. "A Ten-year Follow-up Study of Treated Psychiatric Patients," in AN EVALUATION OF THE RESULTS OF THE PSYCHOTHERAPIES, S. Lesse, Ed. (Springfield, Ill.: Charles C Thomas, 1968).

49. W.L. Kirtner & D.S. Cartwright. Success and Failure in Client-centered Therapy as a Function of Client Personality Variables, *Journal of Consulting Psychology* 22 (1958): 259.

50. W. Janke & G. Debus. "Experimental Studies on Anti-anxiety Agents with Normal Subjects: Methodological Considerations and Review of the Main Effects," in PSYCHOPHARMACOLOGY: A REVIEW OF PROGRESS, 1957-1967, D.H. Efron, Ed. PHS Pub. No. 1836 (Washington, D.C.: Govt. Ptg. Ofc., 1968).

51. E.H. Uhlenhuth, L. Covi & R.S. Lipman. "Indications for Minor Tranquilizers in Anxious Outpatients," in DRUGS AND THE BRAIN, P. Black, Ed. (Baltimore, Md.: John Hopkins Press, 1969).

52. D.M. McNair, R.J. Kahn, L.F. Droppleman & S. Fisher. "Patient Acquiescence and Drug Effects," in NONSPECIFIC FACTORS IN DRUG THERAPY, K. Rickels, Ed. (Springfield, Ill.: Charles C Thomas, 1968).

53. K. Rickels, C.H. Ward & L. Schut. Different Populations, Different Drug Responses: Comparative Study of Two Anti-depressants, Each Used in Two Different Patient Groups, *American Journal of Medical Science*, 247 (1964): 328.

54. G.H. Grosser. "Social and Cultural Considerations in the Treatment of Depression," in PHARMACOTHERAPY OF DEPRESSION, J.O. Cole & J.R. Wittenborn, Eds. (Springfield, Ill.: Charles C Thomas, 1966).

55. J.R. Wittenborn. "Factors Which Qualify the Responses to Iproniazid and Imipramine," in PREDICTION OF RESPONSE TO PHARMACOTHERAPY, J.R. Wittenborn & P.R.A. May, Eds. (Springfield, Ill.: Charles C Thomas, 1966).

56. _____. "Prediction of the Individual's Response to Anti-depressant Medication," in PSYCHOPHARMACOLOGY: A REVIEW OF PROGRESS, 1957-1967, D.H. Efron, Ed. PHS Pub. No. 1836 (Washington, D.C.: Govt. Ptg. Ofc., 1968).

57. J.D. Frank. PERSUASION AND HEALING (Baltimore, Md.: Johns Hopkins University Press, 1961).

58. A.P. Goldstein. THERAPIST-PATIENT EXPECTANCIES IN PSYCHOTHERAPY (New York: MacMillan, 1962).

59. H.J. Friedman. Patient-Expectancy and Symptom Reduction, *Archives of General Psychiatry* 8 (1963): 61.

60. M.D. Sabshin & S.B. Eisen. The Effects of Ward Tension on the Quality and Quantity of Tranquilizer Utilization, *Annals of the New York Academy of Science* 67 (1957): 746.

61. L.A. Gottschalk, G.C. Gleser & W.N. Stone. "Studies of Psychoactive Drug Effects on Nonpsychiatric Patients. Measurement of Affective and Cognitive Changes by Content Analysis of speech," in PSYCHOPHARMACOLOGY OF THE NORMAL HUMAN, W. Evans & N. Kline, Eds. (Springfield, Ill.: Charles C Thomas, 1968).

62. S. Fisher, J.D. Cole, K. Rickels & E.H. Uhlenhuth. Drug-set Interaction: the Effect of Expectations on Drug Response in Outpatients, *Neuropsychopharmacology* 3 (1964): 149.

63. S.G. Kellam, S.C. Goldberg, N.R. Schooler, A. Berman & J.L. Shmelzer. Ward Atmosphere and Outcome of Treatment of Acute Schizophrenia, *Journal of Psychiatric Research* 5 (1967): 145.

64. K. Rickels, R.B. Cattell, A. MacAfee & P. Hesbacher. Drug Response and Important External Events in the Patient's Life, *Diseases of the Nervous System* 26 (1965): 782.

65. L. Bellak & J.B. Chassan. An Approach to the Evaluation of Drug Effect During Psychotherapy: A Double-blind Study of a Single Case, *Journal of Nervous & Mental Disease* 139 (1964): 20.

66. L.A. Gottschalk, F.T. Kapp, W.D. Ross, S.M. Kaplan, H. Silver, J.A. MacLeod, J.B. Kalm, Jr., E.F. Van Maanen & G.H. Acheson. Explorations in Testing Drugs Affecting Physical and Mental Activity, *Journal of the American Medical Association* 161 (1956): 1054.

67. G.C. Gleser, L.A. Gottschalk, R. Fox & W. Lippert. Immediate Changes in Affect with Chlordiazepoxide in Juvenile Delinquent Boys, *Archives of General Psychiatry* 13 (1965): 291.

68. A. Di Francesco. Diazepam, a New Tranquilizer, *American Journal of Psychiatry* 119 (1963): 988.

69. R.J. Kerry & F.A. Jenner. A Double-Blind Crossover Comparison of Diazepam (Valium; R05-2807) with Chlordiazepoxide

(Librium) in the Treatment of Neurotic Anxiety, *Psychopharmacologia* 3 (1962): 302.

70. L.A. Gottschalk, H.W. Elliot, D.E. Bates & C.G. Cable. The Use of Content Analysis of Short Samples of Speech for Preliminary Investigation of Psychoactive Drugs: Effect of Lorazepam on Anxiety Scores, *Clinical Pharmacology & Therapeutics* 13 (1972): 323.

71. W.D. Ross, N. Adsett, G.C. Gleser, C.R.B. Joyce, S.M. Kaplan & M.E. Tieger. A Trial of Psychopharmacologic Measurement with Projective Techniques, *Journal of Projective Techniques* 27 (1963): 223.

72. L.A. Gottschalk, G.C. Gleser, H.W. Wylie, Jr. & S.M. Kaplan. Effects of Imipramine on Anxiety and Hostility Levels Derived from Verbal Communications, *Psychopharmacologia* 7 (1965): 303.

73. W. Nesselhof, D.M. Gallant & M.P. Bishop. A Double-blind Comparison of WY-3498, Diazepam and Placebo in Psychiatric Outpatients, *American Journal of Psychiatry* 121 (1965): 809.

74. M. Lorr, D.M. McNair, G.J. Weinstein, W.W. Michaux & A. Raskin. Meprobamate and Chlorpromazine in Psychotherapy: Some Effects on Anxiety and Hostility of Outpatients, *Archives of General Psychiatry* 4 (1961): 381.

75. M. Lorr, D.M. McNair & G.J. Weinstein. Early Effects of Chlordiazepoxide (Librium) Used with Psychotherapy, *Journal of Psychiatric Research* 1 (1963): 257.

76. I. Roth, P.J. Rhudick, D.A. Shaskan, M.S. Slobin, A.E. Wilkinson & H.H. Young. Long-Term Effects on Psychotherapy of Initial Treatment Conditions, *Journal of Psychiatric Research* 2 (1964): 283.

77. K. Rickels. "Drugs in the Treatment of Neurotic Anxiety and Tension: Controlled Studies," in PSYCHIATRIC DRUGS, P. Solomon, Ed. (New York: Grune & Stratton, 1966).

78. K. Rickels, R.B. Cattell, C. Weise, B. Gray, R. Yee, A. Mallin & H.G. Aaronson. Controlled Psychopharmacological Research in Private Psychiatric Practice, *Psychopharmacologia* 9 (1966): 288.

79. J.D. Frank, L.H. Gliedman, S.D. Imber, A.A. Stone & E.H. Nash. Patients' Expectancies and Relearning as Factors Deter-

mining Improvement in Psychotherapy, *American Journal of Psychiatry* 115 (1959): 961.

80. K. Rickels & R.B. Cattell. "Drug and Placebo Response as a Function of Doctor and Patient Type," in PSYCHOTROPIC DRUG RESPONSE: ADVANCES IN PREDICTION, P.R.A. May & J.R. Wittenborn, Eds. (Springfield, Ill.: Charles C Thomas, 1968).

81. J.R. Wittenborn. THE CLINICAL PHARMACOLOGY OF ANXIETY (Springfield, Ill.: Charles C Thomas, 1966).

82. J.B. Chassan. RESEARCH DESIGN IN CLINICAL PSYCHOLOGY AND PSYCHIATRY (New York: Appleton-Century-Crofts, 1967).

83. B.E. McLaughlin, J.B. Chassan & F. Ryan. Three Single Case Studies Comparing Diazepam and Meprobamate: An Application of Intensive Design, *Comprehensive Psychiatry* 6 (1965): 128.

84. M.A. Jacobs, G. Globus & E. Heim. Reduction in Symptomatology in Ambulatory Patients, *Archives of General Psychiatry* 15 (1966): 45.

# 3

## PHARMACOTHERAPY AND PSYCHOTHERAPY OF SCHIZOPHRENIA

### Studies from the literature

In a study of 80 schizophrenic patients during their first admission to a state hospital, May and Tuma[1] compared the effects of (1) individual psychotherapy two or more hours weekly, (2) trifluoperazine at an individualized dosage, (3) both treatments and (4) neither treatment. Their criteria included discharge rates, length of hospital stay, the adjunctive use of sedation and hydrotherapy, and ratings on the Menninger Health-Sickness Scale. In almost every respect, patients treated with psychotherapy alone responded about the same as the control group whereas patients treated with the drug and the combined treatments during hospitalization responded about the same or significantly better than those receiving psychotherapy alone or the control groups. According to a formal analysis, the variation in outcome was almost entirely due to the drug component of the treatment. Patients treated with drug and psychotherapy combined, however, required somewhat lower doses of the drug than patients treated with the drug alone and had a slightly lower mean stay in the hospital. Neither drug requirement nor duration of stay was statistically significant between the two groups.

In a report by May[2] on the total sample of 228 patients in the same study, similar results were obtained, and the author suggests in his concluding discussion that although "psychotherapy plus drug" was slightly superior to "drug alone," the differences "were often tiny or trivial and never impressive."

61

The lack of immediate demonstrable psychotherapeutic effect in these studies may indicate that severely schizophrenic patients are not very responsive to psychotherapy. The authors have not neglected the rather subtle question of the individual therapist's talent and skill, although it is possible that their therapists' range of skills does not cover the most skilled or gifted. Nonetheless, it does cover the range of skills and experience customarily available. Psychotherapy was provided by state hospital psychiatrists with less than 5 years of experience, including residency. Therapists were not classified as to presumed effectiveness on any other basis in the analyses of results. Real psychotherapeutic effects produced by more competent therapists could therefore have been "washed out" by the failures of less competent therapists. Similar questions arise in some of the other studies reviewed here.

Many observers have suggested that psychotherapy for schizophrenia may have delayed effects that do not become apparent until after discharge from hospital, when they could influence the patient's interpersonal relations and social adjustment. Unfortunately, there are no systematic studies available which would confirm or exclude such a possibility.

Grinspoon et al[3] described a long-term study of 20 chronic schizophrenic patients. Ten were treated with intensive individual psychotherapy by mature therapists, intensive milieu therapy, and placebo; 10 were treated with the same interpersonal treatments and thioridazine, with occasional control periods of placebo. Two behavioral scales and anecdotal material from patients' diaries were used as criteria of change. As measured by all these criteria, the close correlation between the patients' clinical improvement status and the use of thioridazine in their regimen was striking. Reduction in florid symptomatology may have made patients more receptive to the psychotherapist. The interpersonal therapies alone, however, were found to produce no noticeable effects during hospitalization over time.

Other studies in which group therapy was combined with the use of major tranquilizers have yielded similar results. Cowden et al[4] treated four groups of 8 chronic schizophrenic patients for 6 months with (1) ordinary ward management, (2) reserpine at an individually adjusted dosage, (3) placebo plus group psychotherapy 3 hours per week, and (4) reserpine plus group psychotherapy. Criteria of change were constructed from a behavioral rating scale completed by attendants before and after treatment, and tallies of several concrete indices of disturbed behavior before and during the period of treatment—wet packs, seclusion, fights, nurses' reports, ward transfers, and discharge. The attendants' ratings showed no clear differences in response among the four treatment groups. The concrete behavioral indices, however, indicated that the three treated groups responded about the same as or much better than the untreated group, which showed no change.

Interpretation of the results is complicated, first, by the apparent absence of tests for significance of the differences in outcome among the four treatment conditions. Perhaps more important is a defect in design: Group 1 received no placebo. The observed results, therefore, could be partly or wholly due to the act of taking pills, irrespective of their contents, in Groups 2, 3 and 4.

Cowden et al[5] treated three groups of 8 chronic schizophrenic patients for 4 months with (1) ordinary ward management, (2) chlorpromazine at an individually adjusted dosage, and (3) chlorpromazine plus group psychotherapy 3 hours per week. Criteria of change were similar to those described in the preceding study. The two chlorpromazine-treated groups showed greater improvement than the control group on most measures, but the difference in response of the two treated groups was equivocal.

This study incorporates the same defect in design as the previous study; in addition, there is no assessment of the effect of group psychotherapy alone. Consequently, it is impossible to ascertain whether the results in Group 3 are due to ineffective psychotherapy or to interaction between psychotherapy and medication.

King[6] treated five matched groups of 19 chronic schizophrenic patients for 6 months with (1) regressive ECT (RECT), two treatments daily for 11 days; (2) RECT, followed 5 weeks after onset by group psychotherapy once weekly; (3) chlorpromazine, 100 mgm. tid; (4) chlorpromazine, followed 5 weeks after onset by weekly group psychotherapy; and (5) none of these treatments. The criterion of change was a scale composed of psychotic symptoms, with little emphasis on the hyperactivity dimension. The author rated each patient on the scale before and after treatment. Group 1 became significantly worse and Groups 2 and 5 showed no change, while Groups 3 and 4 improved significantly, with Group 4 showing somewhat greater improvement than Group 3. Unfortunately, statistical analyses comparing mean outcomes in the five treatment groups were not given.

King[7] also treated two matched groups of 20 chronic schizophrenic women each for one year with (1) chlorpromazine, 100 mgm. tid, and (2) chlorpromazine plus weekly group psychotherapy. Six months after termination of group psychotherapy, 7 patients who had had chlorpromazine alone and 6 patients who had had combined treatment were discharged in complete remission. The author concluded that group psychotherapy offered no benefit beyond that of the drug. The experimental design of the study and the single criterion of change seriously restrict the conclusions that can be drawn from it.

Evangelakis[8] treated five matched groups of 20 chronically hospitalized patients for 4 to 18 months with (1) placebo plus in-ward and off-ward activities plus group psychotherapy twice weekly; (2) trifluoperazine at an individually adjusted dosage; (3) trifluoperazine plus in-ward activities; (4) trifluoperazine plus off-ward activities; and (5) trifluoperazine plus in-ward and off-ward activities plus group psychotherapy. His criteria of improvement included ward transfers and various types of discharge. He found that patients responded poorly to the social therapies alone (Group 1), better to trifluoperazine alone (Group 2), and still better to the social therapies combined with trifluoperazine (Groups 3, 4 and 5). Off-ward activities appeared to be the most effective component of the social therapies.

In this study, interpretation of the interaction between treatments again is uncertain, because the effects of the various treatments alone are not adequately assessed. In particular the nature of the group therapy is not made clear. Obviously, group psychotherapy in this and other studies of psychotic patients in continuous contact on a ward in a large hospital may have very little in common with dynamically oriented group psychotherapy as practiced with psychoneurotic patients in an office setting.

Honigfeld et al[9] reported a large, VA multihospital study of 256 chronic schizophrenic men aged 54-74, treated for 24 weeks in eight groups with (1), individualized doses of acetophenazine, imipramine, trifluoperazine, or placebo, plus social group therapy twice weekly; or (2), individualized dosages of one of the three drugs used in the study, or placebo, without group therapy. Criteria of change were based on the Inpatient Multidimensional Psychiatric Scale and the Nurses' Observation Scale for Inpatient Evaluation.

Patients who received acetophenazine or trifluoperazine generally improved more than patients who received other medications. Patients who participated in group therapy generally improved more than patients who did not participate. The authors stated that the treatments showed neither "joint effects" nor "additive effects." Their findings seemed to suggest that the effects of the combined treatments were about the same as the effects of the medications or the group psychotherapy separately, but they were presented in a way that makes it impossible to clarify this point.

In another VA cooperative study, Gorham et al[10] studied 150 relatively acute schizophrenic men treated with (1) 36 sessions of group psychotherapy, 3 hours per week; (2) thioridazine, 300-500 mgm. daily for 12 weeks; or (3) both treatments combined. Their criteria of change consisted of five global measures and the Brief Psychiatric Rating Scale (BPRS). All global measures showed that the groups receiving drug alone or combined treatment responded about the same as and significantly better than the group receiving group psychotherapy alone. Most of the BPRS scale ratings gave the same result.

Similar studies yielding substantially the same conclusions have been reported by others.[11-13]

## Clinical significance of studies reviewed

The studies cited are quite diverse in design and methods, but they share enough common ground to reveal several trends. In the treatment of schizophrenic patients with medication and group psychotherapy, two studies suggest that combined treatment is superior to psychotherapy alone and two early studies suggest that combined treatment offers no advantage during hospitalization over group therapy alone. However, one of these early studies used reserpine and another used low doses of chlorpromazine.

Three studies suggest that combined treatment is superior to drug treatment alone and five studies suggest that combined treatment offers no clear advantage over drugs alone. In short, there is no clear evidence that adding group psychotherapy to medication offers additional benefit for schizophrenic patients.

In the treatment of schizophrenic patients with medication and individual psychotherapy, two studies suggest that combined treatment is superior to psychotherapy alone and one study suggests that combined treatment is not superior to drug treatment alone. In other words, very few of the reported studies address themselves directly to a comparison of treatment outcomes from psychotherapy and pharmacotherapy—alone and in combination—with schizophrenics. In addition, methodological weaknesses in several of the studies reviewed make it difficult to draw firm inferences.

The weight of current evidence indicates that adding individual psychotherapy to medication offers little if any additional benefit for schizophrenic patients during hospitalization. Many more well-designed comparative studies of various treatments and their combinations seem essential. It is lamentable that major public health decisions about the treatment of schizophrenia are being made on the basis of pitifully few studies, and that decisions on educational and treatment programs are not being made on a scientific basis.

In the face of this situation and despite the early admonitions of Freud that the psychoses and the narcissistic neuroses are not amenable to psychoanalysis, there are a number of dedicated psychoanalysts who report dramatic recoveries with psychoanalytic therapy (e.g., Laing, Arieti, Will, Searles). These cases are few in number and the practical limitations of the treatment precluding its widespread use mean that it can have little impact on the massive social problems occasioned by the high incidence of schizophrenia. Nonetheless, were it possible to establish a successful psychotherapy for schizophrenia, this would raise important theoretical questions concerning the nature of the illness.

Whitehorn and Betz,[14] in a study of the exclusively psychological treatment of primarily acute schizophrenia, correlated patient improvement rates with personal characteristics and therapeutic strategies of individual therapists, all of whom had comparable clinical experience. The results showed that high improvement rates were correlated with treatment strategies (Group A physicians) which emphasized active patient-physician interaction generating confidence and rapport, insight into problem areas and capabilities for their constructive resolution, and an attitude of respect for the patient as an individual—including a willingness to disagree with him in a rational, non-authoritarian manner. Low improvement rates, on the other hand, were found to be correlated with treatment strategies (Group B physicians) emphasizing a less personal relationship and fewer directive measures, a passive-permissive attitude toward the patient, and treatment goals that were primarily pathology-oriented, such as symptom reduction and "increased socialization." Other studies have yielded a mixture of findings, some supporting and some contradicting early conclusions.

More recently, Karon and O'Grady[15] and Karon and Vanden Bos[16] have reported results from a study in which 36 schizophrenics were randomly assigned to a group receiving (A) "active" psychoanalytic therapy, (B) psychoanalytic therapy of an "ego-analytic" variety using medication adjunctively, or (C) medication plus supportive psychotherapy. Groups A and B were further subdivided into patients treated by senior clinical supervisors or by student therapists (graduate students in clinical psychology and psychiatric residents). Evaluations of 6-month treatment schedules showed that although both Groups A and B improved more than Group C, there were significant differences in the improvement rates of patients treated by the experienced senior therapists compared to those treated by the residents and graduate students. The authors conclude that senior therapist-treated patient improvement rates were comparable in both Groups A and B regardless of medication, and that the addition of medication showed a significantly positive effect only for those Group B patients treated by the inexperienced student therapists. The authors refer specifically to the 1964 May and Tuma study reviewed above[1] and suggest that its conclusions are "consistent with our findings for the inexperienced therapists, but not for the supervisors." Karon and

Vanden Bos[16] criticize them for reporting data only on patients treated by inexperienced therapists (psychiatric residents under supervision). These authors go on to say, "It would seem that the use of medication is most important to the inexperienced therapist." However, since their patients were not randomly assigned to experienced and inexperienced therapists, their data are not convincing.

The Whitehorn and Betz study[14] was conducted before psychotropic drugs were available, and although their patient population is not clearly defined, it is likely that it was comprised mainly of acute schizophrenic reactions. Both the Karon and O'Grady study[15] and the subsequent Karon and Vanden Bos report[16] appear to have serious methodological faults and are written in a fashion that makes interpretation difficult.

Furthermore, the general implication that experienced psychotherapists do not need to use drugs is contrary to the findings of Grinspoon *et al* in whose study the experience of the psychotherapists was quite extensive; and even to those of May,[2] in whose study therapists had as much as six years of experience and received weekly supervision by psychoanalysts experienced in the treatment of schizophrenic patients.

Insofar as the conclusions of Karon and associates are contrary to the other reports available in the literature, they must be considered carefully. Although the authors' conclusions are at variance with those of the May study, close scrutiny of the design and statistical analyses prompts many questions about the appropriateness of the methods employed and the conclusions drawn.[17] Yet they are clearly in accord with the conviction of some clinicians that prolonged intensive psychotherapy is the treatment of choice in schizophrenia, at least for patients whose symptomatology is not so florid or advanced toward chronicity as to render them totally inaccessible to interpersonal and interpretive methods.

Clearly, there is room for significant improvement in the

treatment of schizophrenia. Before ataractics, follow-up studies revealed that approximately 30-40% of acute schizophrenics recover and stay well or much improved for periods of 5 to 20 years.[18-21] Since the advent of the major psychotropic drugs, the picture has not changed in an entirely satisfactory way. Despite high initial discharge rates, relapses are common and occur much more frequently when drugs are discontinued.[22-25] The optimum social environment for the discharged schizophrenic seems to be a stable and emotionally secure climate with significant cognitive input.[22] It is difficult to believe that a type of psychotherapy or sociotherapy which would engender that kind of stability would have no role in the prevention of relapses in the schizophrenia patient.

In the face of existing evidence, it is impossible to believe that chronic or intermittent use of drugs, perhaps to stabilize the internal environment of the schizophrenic patient, is not without considerable value in continued treatment. Without drugs, relapse rates in the first year are 40% or higher; for conscientious drug takers, the rate is still 20%.[26] Thus, more research is needed both on drug usage and on the various forms of psychotherapy and sociotherapy before we can hope to improve treatment substantially.

## References

1. P.R.A. May & A.H. Tuma. The Effect of Psychotherapy and Stelazine on Length of Hospital Stay, Release Rate and Supplemental Treatment of Schizophrenic Patients, *Journal of Nervous & Mental Disease* 139 (1964): 362.
2. P.R.A. May. TREATMENT OF SCHIZOPHRENIA (New York: Science House, 1968).
3. L. Grinspoon, J.R. Ewalt & R. Shader. Psychotherapy and Pharmacotherapy in Chronic Schizophrenia, *American Journal of Psychiatry* 124 (1968): 1645.
4. R.C. Cowden, M. Zax & J.A. Sproles. Reserpine Alone and as an Adjunct to Psychotherapy in the Treatment of Schizophrenia,

*American Medical Association Archives of Neurology & Psychiatry* 74 (1955): 518.

5. R.C. Cowden, M. Zax, J.R. Hague & R.C. Finney. Chlorpromazine: Alone and as an Adjunct to Group Psychotherapy in the Treatment of Psychiatric Patients, *American Journal of Psychiatry* 112 (1956): 898.

6. P.D. King. Regressive ECT, Chlorpromazine, and Group Therapy in Treatment of Hospitalized Chronic Schizophrenics, *American Journal of Psychiatry* 115 (1958): 354.

7. _____. Controlled Study of Group Psychotherapy in Schizophrenics Receiving Chlorpromazine, *Psychiatric Digest* 24 (1963): 21.

8. M.G. Evangelakis. De-institutionalization of Patients: The Triad of Trifluoperazine - Group Psychotherapy - Adjunctive Therapy, *Diseases of the Nervous System* 22 (1961): 26.

9. G. Honigfeld, M.P. Rosenblum, I.J. Blumenthal, H.L. Lambert & A.J. Roberts. Behavioral Improvement in the Older Schizophrenic Patient: Drug and Social Therapies, *Journal of the American Geriatric Society* 13 (1964): 57.

10. D.R. Gorham, A.D. Pokorny, E.C. Moseley, P. McRenolds & W.S. Kogan. Effects of a Phenothiazine and/or Group Psychotherapy with Schizophrenics, *Diseases of the Nervous System* 25 (1964): 77.

11. R.I. Shader, L. Grinspoon, J.R. Ewalt & D.A. Zahn. "Drug Responses in Acute Schizophrenia," in SCHIZOPHRENIA—AN APPRAISAL (Hicksville, N.Y.: P.J.D. Publishers) in press.

12. J.J. Gibbs, B. Wilkens & C.G. Lauterbach. A Controlled Clinical Psychiatric Study of Chlorpromazine, *Journal of Clinical & Experimental Psychopathology* 18 (1957): 269.

13. R.S. Bookhammer, R.W. Meyers, C.C. Schober & Z.A. Piotrowski. A Five Year Clinical Follow-up Study of Schizophrenics Treated by Rosen's "Direct Analysis" Compared with Controls, *American Journal of Psychiatry* 123 (1966): 602.

14. J.C. Whitehorn & B.J. Betz. A Study of Psychotherapeutic Relationships Between Physicians and Schizophrenic Patients, *American Journal of Psychiatry* 11 (1954): 321.

15. B.P. Karon & P. O'Grady. Intellectual Test Changes in Schizophrenic Patients in the First Six Months of Treatment, *Psychotherapy: Theory, Research & Practice* 6 (1969): 88.

16. B.P. Karon & G.R. Vanden Bos. Experience, Medication, and the Effectiveness of Psychotherapy with Schizophrenics, *British Journal of Psychiatry* 116 (1970): 427.
17. P.R.A. May & A.H. Tuma. Methodological Problems in Psychotherapy Research, *British Journal of Psychiatry* 117 (1970): 569.
18. K.E. Appel, J.M. Myers & A.E. Scheflen. Prognosis in Psychiatry: Results of Psychiatric Treatment, *AMA Archives of Neurology. & Psychiatry* 70 (1953): 459.
19. C. Astrup, A. Fossum & R. Holmboe. PROGNOSIS IN FUNCTIONAL PSYCHOSES (Springfield, Ill.: Charles C Thomas, 1963).
20. W. Malamud & N. Render. Course and Prognosis in Schizophrenia, *American Journal of Psychiatry* 95 (1939): 1039.
21. T.A.C. Rennie. Follow-up Study of 500 Patients with Schizophrenia Admitted to Hospital from 1913 to 1923, *AMA Archives of Neurology & Psychiatry* 42 (1939): 877.
22. J. Wing, J. Leff & S. Hirsch. "Preventive Treatment of Schizophrenia: Some Theoretical and Methodological Issues." Paper presented at a meeting of the APPA, New York, New York, March 4, 1972.
23. S.C. Goldberg, J.O. Cole & G.L. Klerman. "Differential Prediction of Improvement Under 3 Phenothiazines," in PREDICTION OF RESPONSE TO PHARMACOTHERAPY, J.R. Wittenborn & P.R.A. May, Eds. (Springfield, Ill.: Charles C Thomas, 1966).
24. R. Gittelman-Klein & D. Klein. "Long-term Effects of 'Antipsychotic' Agents: A Review," in PSYCHOPHARMACOLOGY: A REVIEW OF PROGRESS 1957-1967, D.H. Efron, Ed. PHS Pub. No. 1836 (Washington, D.C.: U.S. Govt. Ptg. Ofc., 1968), page 1119.
25. R.F. Prien & C.J. Klett. An Appraisal of the Long-term Use of Tranquilizing Medication with Hospitalized Chronic Schizophrenics: A Review of Drug Discontinuation Literature, *Schizophrenia Bulletin* No. 5 (1972).
26. G.E. Hogarty & S.C. Goldberg. Drug and Sociotherapy in the post Hospital Maintenance of Schizophrenic Patients: One Year Relapse Rates, *AMA Archives of General Psychiatry*, 1972.

# 4

## PHARMACOTHERAPY AND PSYCHOTHERAPY OF DEPRESSION

Depression is the most common of the major psychiatric syndromes, with perhaps 10 per cent of the United States population having an episode of clinical depression at some point in their lives.[1] It is also among the syndromes most actively researched. Several excellent books, monographs and papers have been published which summarize the present state of the art with respect to its genetics,[2,3] the influence of early environmental experiences,[4,5] the problems involved in classification,[6,7] its psychodynamics,[8,9] its behavioral characteristics,[10] and its neurobiology.[11,12] Useful hypotheses regarding the role of the chemical transmitter systems in the biology of depression have been offered.[13]

Depression does not seem to be unique to the human species but can be generated in some animals, thus offering the possibility for further investigation with a degree of freedom not available in studies on man.[14-16]

Remarkable changes have occurred in the clinical treatment of depression with the introduction and acceptance of ECT, monoamine oxidase (MAO) inhibitors, and especially the tricyclic antidepressants and lithium.[7,17-19] Research combining neuroendocrinology with pharmacology is also very active and offers promise of accelerating the treatment and improving the efficacy of treatment for drug-resistant patients.[20,21]

Although clinical practice in treatment of depression has altered, our basic concepts underlying the psychotherapy of depressions remain unchanged. Even though antidepressant and tranquilizing drugs are now frequently prescribed as adjuncts to the psychotherapy of depression, few attempts have been made to integrate the available neurobiological findings into currently accepted clinical concepts of the psychogenesis and psychotherapy of depression.

In this chapter, the psychodynamic and neurochemical models of depression are discussed, not by way of a comprehensive review, but rather in a critical summary of these two models calculated to highlight the relationship of the psychodynamic and neurochemical models at the theoretical level, and to provide a potential working rationale for clinical practice. Thus, important aspects of the overall problem of the genetics of depression will not be covered, and little will be said about the role of familial structure and early environmental experiences, particularly those resulting from parental loss and separation.

## PROTOTHEORIES AND MODELS

Depression serves as a paradigm of the compartmentalized and fragmented state of contemporary psychiatric thought. The issues raised in depression apply equally to other clinical states but are examined here as a specific illustration of general problems. This fragmentation can be understood as an example of "cognitive dissonance," the concept developed by Festinger. Faced with a lack of congruence between their clinical practices and theoretical rationales, practitioners tend to utilize partial theories, which we shall call "prototheories," that are as a rule not worked out or articulated explicitly. Conceptual issues are frequently avoided and theoretical concerns are separated from actual clinical practice.

The clinician's selection of drugs and/or psychotherapy is usually based on his training and therapeutic orientation, his empirical experience, and his pragmatic goals. Research data and theoretical aims are seldom foremost in therapeutic decision-making, yet various concepts, formulations and methodological commitments are implicit in this process. Such a treatment rationale is usually the manifest expression of an implicit theoretical model.[22]

If we ask clinicians to explain their rationale for prescribing various therapies, we can readily discern conflicting ideas. Thus, if we ask a psychotherapist why he uses a particular psychotherapeutic technique, he will almost always answer in terms of psychodynamic concepts—resolution of conflict, change of personality structure, and reduction of depression. Now, if we ask a psychotherapist why he prescribes drugs, he will seldom answer in psychodynamic terms. Rather he will discuss the patient's reduction of symptoms, perhaps noting that drugs facilitate psychotherapy, but he will probably be vague about the processes by which the drug facilitates treatment.

Prototheories are rationales which underlie and justify the nature of working decisions made by practitioners. A prototheory exemplifies an ideological rationale. As such, a prototheory is subject not only to intellectual discussion and scientific verification, but is understandable as the mode by which professionals explain their ideological commitments and treatment decisions to themselves, each other, and the larger public. Thus, the prototheory serves both as a justification of the treatment decision process and as a presumed scientific explanation of the basis for clinical practice. It may well be that in the development of scientific theory in psychiatry, theoretical ideas lag behind practice. Clearly this is true in most therapeutic practice in which empirical evidence often guides clinicians to a far greater extent than the data available from systematic clinical trials and experimental studies.

## The psychodynamic model of depression

The classic psychodynamic model of depression derives from the early 20th century observations of Abraham[23] and Freud.[24] A summary of psychoanalytic contributions is offered by Beck[6] who discusses the work of Rado, Gero, Bibring, Klein, Jacobson and Zeitzel. Based upon their observations of similarities and differences between clinical depression and normal bereavement, these workers hypothesized the psychodynamic importance of actual or fantasied loss as a precipitant of clinical depression. Clinical depression involves a regression to oral-sadistic levels, a regression precipitated by the patient's guilt and aggression due to his difficulties in relinquishing his libidinal ties to a lost object.

Predisposition to depression is caused by a number of factors: constitutional determinants of oral drive strength; early childhood trauma, particularly trauma resulting in fixations in the late oral and early anal libidinal phases; and the development of an adult personality organized around rigid ego defenses, a strong superego, the inhibition of expression of aggression, strong dependency wishes, narcissistic object relations, and difficulties in relinquishing object ties.

The acute depressive illness may be precipitated by an actual loss, but more frequently by a situational change which has the unconscious meaning to the patient of significant loss.[25] During clinical depression, the bereaved and aggrieved patient's defenses against hostility and guilt intensify as he grapples with his rage toward the internalized object of identification. In this classic view, the clinical features of depression emerge from the struggle between two psychic structures, the ego and the superego. Clinical manifestations of agitation, self-deprecation, guilt, inhibition of ego functions, and suicidal drive are understood in terms of these dynamic and structural concepts.

In recent decades, ego psychology and sociocultural studies have proposed significant alternatives to this classical theory. Within psychoanalysis, many ego psychologists now view the psychogenesis of depression as the ego's response to fluctuations in self-esteem. Bibring developed a comprehensive formulation in which depression is described as an ego state capable of emerging independently of the dynamics of aggression or of libidinal drives. Developments in ego psychology have deemphasized the ego conflict, regarding depression as an affect similar to anxiety in its adaptive function.[8,26,27]

The sociocultural point of view, first noted in Durkheim's sociological and anthropological research on suicide in the 1890's, emphasizes environmental factors and stresses the importance of ethnic identity and social class. Linkages between the sociocultural view and the ego psychological approach can be seen in the family background studies of depressives by Mabel Blake Cohen and her associates[28] and by Gibson,[29] who emphasizes the marginality of the depressive's family of origin and the dependent nature of his interpersonal relations, even in the nondepressed phase.

As Mendelson[9] and Beck[6] have emphasized, and as shown in the preceding discussion, there is as yet no single comprehensive model in contemporary psychiatric theory for the psychogenesis and psychodynamics of depression. If anything, there appear to be alternative and at times competing complementary viewpoints.

## The introduction of drugs into the psychotherapy of depression

Although drugs are now prescribed for the treatment of depression by psychiatrists of all persuasions, the dynamically oriented psychotherapist usually considers them to be adjuncts to the psychotherapy of depression. Usually, such physicians claim that drugs reduce manifest symptoms and relieve the subjective distress of the patient. Prominent symptoms, such as anxiety, insomnia, tension and visceral manifestations, are the target symptoms of drug prescription. The physician attempts to alleviate the patient's subjective distress in order to facilitate communication, to reduce resistance to therapeutic insight, and to accelerate psychotherapeutic progress. This current widespread use of drugs in combination with psychotherapy in the treatment of depression raises complex issues related to the mind-body problem in psychiatry and medicine. Theoretically, studies of the actions of antidepressant drugs involve the possible relationship of CNS substrates to affect, ego functions, and symptom formation. Here, two areas of research would seem to have the greatest potential value:

**1. Studies of the efficacy of combined psychotherapy and drug therapy.** As indicated, it is now uncommon to find a severely depressed patient who receives psychotherapy but is not given medication to assist sleep, reduce anxiety, or relieve depression. Similarly, it is uncommon for patients on drug therapy not to receive some form of psychotherapy as well, even if it is only supportive counseling and reassurance. However, there is as yet little systematic empirical evidence supporting the efficacy of this combination. Are there antagonisms between drugs and psychotherapy? Do drugs really facilitate psychotherapeutic communication? Does a too rapid amelioration of symptoms impair the patient's motivation for insight? These and similar questions require controlled empirical validation for answer.

**2. Studies of the psychodynamic effects of drug treatment.** Drug therapy produces significant changes, not only in target symptoms, but also in psychodynamic functioning. Ostow[30] has interpreted drug effects in terms of psychoanalytic libidinal theory. Such psychoanalysts as Sarwer-Foner,[31] Azima,[32] and Bellak et al[33] have emphasized their effects on various ego functions. The work of Whitman and others in Cincinnati has placed emphasis on changes in dream content. In addition, there have been studies of drug effects on hostility, anxiety and other affects.[34,35] Changes in sleep mechanisms and patterns as a result of drug action have also been the subject of psychodynamic study. Further studies in this area

offer promise of elucidating psychodynamic mechanisms involved in antidepressant drug action; conversely, experimental alterations of CNS amines by pharmacological means
could clarify the role of neurochemical substrates in the
psychodynamics of affect regulation.

Various approaches (prototheories) to antidepressant drug
therapy are implicit in a psychotherapist's decision to use
drugs. These prototheories of depression lend themselves to
an analysis of the psychodynamic and neurochemical models
and to an exploration of the potential for linkages between
these two theoretical orientations. It is hoped that by critical
analyses of these concepts and theories, research can be generated which will contribute to the resolution of the theoretical conflicts between the two models and facilitate further
rational therapeutic planning.

## The neurochemical model of depression

If we were to ask a drug-oriented psychiatrist why he prescribes drugs, he would probably reply that his rationale is
similar in some respects to the psychotherapist's. He expects
drugs to reduce target symptoms, and ultimately to reduce
the patient's subjective distress. In clinical decision-making,
both the psychotherapist and the pharmacotherapist have a
common immediate goal—symptom reduction—but their
long-term goals are usually different. Whereas the psychotherapist views the reduction of distress as facilitating the
constructive new learning engendered by the psychotherapeutic process, the pharmacotherapist tends to see
symptom reduction as primarily facilitating the patient's social adjustment and accelerating spontaneous remission. If
pressed further, the pharmacotherapist may shift from this
aspect of his prototheory to a more complex formulation of
the mode of action of the antidepressant drugs, in
pharmacological and neurochemical terms—citing, for ex-

ample, the recent studies on catecholamines and indoleamines.

Pharmacological studies of the MAO inhibitors and the
tricyclic derivatives have contributed to the development of
the amine hypothesis of affective disorders. In its simplest
form, this hypothesis can be stated as follows: that depression
is accompanied by a functional unavailability of CNS amines,
especially norepinephrine, and can be treated by increasing
them either by inhibition of degradation, as in the case of
MAO inhibitors, or by blockage of membrane uptake, as with
the tricyclic antidepressants.[13]

Although investigators disagree about the relative role of
indoleamines and catecholamines in the pathogenesis of depression, they agree on basic neurophysiological concepts.
Nonetheless, despite the fact that most antidepressant drug
therapy is accompanied by at least minimal psychotherapy,
for the most part amine investigators have been noncommittal
about the etiology and pathogenesis of these presumed dys-
functions in CNS amine metabolism. Some hypothesize that
the predisposition to altered amine metabolism may be a
quantitative deviation from the norm, possibly precipitated by
stress, childhood experience, conditioning, nutrition, or
other vicissitudes of development and experience. A few con-
tend that there are some genetically determined abnor-
malities which have a hereditary-familial basis, and they emphasize the importance to theory of discovered familial patterns in manic-depressive disorders, particularly those with "a
streak of mania."[2,3]

Psychoendocrine studies do help to provide linkages between amine theory and psychodynamic and environmental
factors. Research by Sachar,[36] Bliss et al,[37] and Bunney and
Hamburg and their co-workers[38] substantiates adrenal response to psychic stress in depressive episodes. There is ample
evidence that the adrenal-pituitary system is subtly responsive
to environmental changes and life experiences.

Furthermore, evidence is accumulating that amine metabolism is altered by neuroendocrine states. Consequently, the possibility exists that factors such as acute stress (e.g., grief), conflict, or chronic deprivation may have indirect effects upon amine metabolism. For example, a recent study[39] of infant monkeys in the "protest stage" following separation from their mothers shows marked induction of adrenal catecholamine enzymes. No changes were noted in the brain. Similar studies of the "despair stage" have yet to be done. Furthermore, no work of this kind has been done on human subjects. This possibility therefore remains an hypothesis rather than an established finding.

Stressful episodes like grief and bereavement are normal, expected experiences in life. Yet we know relatively little about their associated psychosomatic aspects. What are the autonomic and other psychophysiological changes in grief? Is the pathophysiology of grief similar to that of depression? Do they only differ in onset, intensity and duration? Is there any rationale for drug therapy during grief? Does the premature relief of distress and grief by therapeutic intervention abort the work of normal mourning and hence predispose the individual to a later depression, as has been hypothesized by Lindemann?[40] There is simply no evidence resolving this issue.

## Competition and cooperation

Theoretically, the neurochemical and psychodynamic models are at different levels of discourse, but ideologically they are usually competitive. Linkages and bridges between the two models are few and at best enjoy tenuous theoretical and empirical support. Although considerable psychophysiological research has been undertaken in animals and man to document the mechanisms by which conflict and stress influence brain function (particularly at pituitary, hypothalamic and subcortical levels), endocrine activity, and amine metabolism, explicit formulations of the use of psychotherapy in pharmacotherapeutic practice are rare. In clinical practice, these models are used simultaneously, although only in eclectic and pragmatic fashion.

It is regrettable that so little attention has been given the interactions between these two therapeutic approaches. At the present time, only a few controlled clinical trials assessing combinations of drugs and psychotherapy have been reported. Thus, Friedman,[41] in an abstract, reports that drug therapy was superior to marital therapy for symptom relief and clinical improvement. Effects of marital therapy were superior to those of drug therapy on the patient's self-rating in family role tasks and on patient perception of the marital relationship.

L. Covi and his co-workers[42,43] noted that imipramine therapy showed a strong advantage over diazepam and placebo. Results of group therapy did not differ reliably from those of minimal contact therapy and imipramine effects were stronger under minimal contact conditions.

Klerman et al[44] recently reported results with 150 neurotic depressed female patients who were treated with amitryptiline and psychotherapy, alone and in combination, for an 8-month period. Amitryptiline with low psychotherapeutic contact resulted in a 12% relapse rate. Placebo with psychotherapy, using an experienced social worker who saw the patients weekly, resulted in a 16% relapse rate. The combination offered no significant alteration in relapse rate over the drug alone. However, psychotherapy did improve social adjustment as measured by improvement in the marital situation, less interpersonal friction, increased communication, and better relations with close family members. The nature of the psychotherapy in this experiment was largely supportive and dealt with here-and-now issues. These studies, though still preliminary, support the value of pharmacotherapy in improving mood and reducing symptoms, but they also suggest that psychotherapy aimed at helping the patient to solve interpersonal problems is of value.

While awaiting further studies, it should prove useful to analyze the possibly competitive and/or cooperative relationships between the two forms of treatment. Our approach to this analysis is to outline the possible interactions when the two forms are combined—to ask: What possible effects (positive and negative) upon the psychotherapeutic process and upon the outcome of treatment can we expect from the introduction of drug therapy? and, conversely, what effects can we expect upon the pharmacotherapeutic process and the outcome of treatment from the introduction of psychotherapy? Although the effects of drugs and psychotherapy upon each other will be discussed only for depression, it will be apparent that similar considerations arise in combined treatments for other disorders.

## Possible negative effects of drug therapy on psychotherapy

Interestingly, most attention has been paid to the possible negative effects upon psychotherapy of introducing drug therapy, and although relatively little empirical research has been done on this problem, it is possible to identify a number of potential effects:

**1) The negative placebo effect.** Much of the criticism of drug therapy voiced by psychotherapists in the 1950's implied a negative placebo effect—that pill-taking had harmful effects on psychotherapy. It was argued that the prescription of drugs had deleterious effects upon the psychotherapeutic relationship and upon the attitudes and behavior of both patient and therapist, effects independent of the specific pharmacological actions of the drug. Presumably the prescription of medications promoted an authoritarian attitude on the part of the psychiatrist and enhanced his belief in his biological-medical heritage, while at the same time, the patient would become more dependent, place greater reliance on magical thinking, and assume a more passive, compliant role, as is expected in the conventional doctor-patient relationship in fields of medicine other than psychiatry.

Thus, the introduction of medication into the psychotherapeutic process was hypothesized as initiating and/or augmenting countertransference and transference processes which militate against the development of insight and the uncovering of defenses. Although insight and uncovering therapy was not specifically used in the Klerman studies, it is nevertheless worth noting that no negative effects of the drug on psychotherapy were noted.[44]

**2) Drug-induced reduction of anxiety and symptoms as motives for discontinuing psychotherapy.** In contrast to the negative placebo effect hypothesis above, which deals only with the symbolic and psychological meaning of drug administration, this objection acknowledges the therapeutic pharmacological actions of drugs, but its proponents express concern that the resultant decrease of anxiety and tension may reduce the patient's motivation for active participation in the psychotherapeutic process. The hypothesis is that too effective a drug will initiate forces countering progress in psychotherapy.

Thus, if a psychoactive drug, such as a phenothiazine or diazepoxide derivative, is very effective in reducing psychotic turmoil, neurotic anxiety or other symptoms, the patient's motivation for reflection, insight, and psychotherapeutic work will be impaired.[45,46] According to this hypothesis, it may be predicted that if drug therapy is "too" effective, patients will no longer seek psychotherapy because they will be satisfied with a reduction of their symptoms and therefore will cease working toward deeper personality and characterological changes. Again, in the few studies which have been reported by Klerman[44] and Covi et al,[42] no evidence was found to support this position.

**3) Pharmacotherapy undercuts defenses.** This hypothesis holds that if the pharmacological effect of a drug prematurely undercuts some important defense, symptom substitution may ensue—compensatory alternative mechanisms of symptom formation. In psychotherapeutic practice, Seitz[47] has reported instances of new symptom formation following hypnosis, and E. Weiss[27] has cautioned against an overly rapid relief of the agoraphobic's anxiety. If his anxiety is reduced too rapidly, before new defenses are developed, other symptoms may emerge. This hypothesis assumes that symptoms maintain the balance between conflict and defenses, and that the precipitous reduction of anxiety, depression or tension may upset this equilibrium and activate deeper conflicts. If so, this would obviously generate new problems for the neurotic or depressive patient, but systematic research data and replications bearing on this specific issue are few and inconclusive.

**4) State-dependent learning.** In animal experiments, Miller[48,49] and Overton[50] have found that with barbiturates, amphetamines and alcohol, new learning may be state-dependent and possibly may not persist upon termination of drug therapy. Since these agents were used in massive doses in the animal studies and do not resemble the major or minor tranquilizers, this limitation is not likely to apply to commonly used psychotropic drugs and human subjects, but it is still important to verify or exclude this possible effect on human beings by further study.

**5) Possible deleterious effects of pharmacotherapy upon psychotherapeutic expectations.** The patient may have a negative reaction when he is prescribed drug therapy, since he may have expected psychotherapy. The patient may feel that the prescription of a drug defines him as "less interesting," as an unsuitable candidate for insight therapy. Thus, the use of drugs may result in a loss of self-esteem on the part of the patient—especially if he belongs to the cultural subgroup

which emphasizes the attainment of insight, psychotherapeutic understanding, and self-actualization. This expectation varies with the subculture of the patient. Within
groups that value psychotherapy, the use of drugs is sometimes regarded as a "failure crutch."

## Possible positive effects of drug therapy on psychotherapy

The five effects described above are postulated as having
negative influences on the psychotherapeutic process. Although these possible negative influences have been given the
closest attention by clinicians, equal consideration must be
given to the possible positive effects through which drug
therapy may facilitate, augment, and interact in a synergistic
manner with individual psychotherapy and other psycho-
social therapies. At least four such effects may be identified:

**1) Drugs facilitate accessibility.** This effect is embodied in the
most commonly held view underlying the use of combined
therapies and is the prototheory which supports the prevail-
ing clinical practice in psychiatry. The advertisements and
other promotional materials of many pharmaceutical firms
propose that introduction of the drug in question will facilitate psychotherapy by making the patient "more accessible."
The mechanism is readily stated—the pharmacological action
of the drug ameliorates the presumptive CNS substrate dysfunction underlying symptom formation, resulting in reduction of the patient's symptomatology, psychopathology,
and/or affective discomfort.

This reduction of discomfort renders the patient better able
to communicate and learn constructively in psychotherapy
—that is, some degree of anxiety, dysphoria or symptomatology is necessary to provide a drive or motivation for psychotherapy. According to this view, high levels of tension, anxiety
or symptom intensity decrease the patient's capacity to participate effectively in psychotherapy. Appropriate use of

drugs is said to permit an optimum level of discomfort needed for psychotherapeutic work.

**2) Drugs enhance the ego psychological functioning required for participation in psychotherapy.** Another mechanism by which it is thought drugs may positively influence the psychotherapeutic process is their pharmacologic action on neurophysiological substrates for the ego functions essential to participation in the psychotherapeutic process. Some drugs may enhance verbal skills, improve cognitive functioning and memory, reduce distractibility, and promote attention and concentration. These psychological functions and abilities are components of the larger domain of ego function, and it is widely accepted that adequate ego functioning is a prerequisite for participation in the psychotherapeutic process.

**3) Abreactive effects.** One of the earliest psychotherapeutic techniques initially described by Breuer and Freud in their studies of hysteria was hypnosis, used to promote catharsis or abreaction. More recently, a number of drugs, especially intravenous barbiturates and amphetamines, have been used to promote this effect. Wikler,[51] in his monograph on the pharmacological basis of psychiatric therapy, referred to such methods as "psychoexploratory techniques." These drugs help to uncover memory, break down defenses, and bring to consciousness material against which the patient otherwise defends. A variant of this practice is the recent use of LSD, mescaline, or psilocybin to promote "peak experiences" in which the heightened sense of self-awareness and the emotional, affective and bodily experiences that occur under the influence of these psychedelic drugs are advocated to facilitate the psychotherapeutic process.

**4) Positive placebo effect on drug therapy.** The advocates of publicly congenial biological methods, such as the megavitamin treatment of schizophrenia, are in effect helping to remove the stigma from psychiatric illness and in some instances are making it easier for the patient to accept the definition of himself as mentally ill. Thus, the request for drug therapy may itself be a vehicle through which the patient can seek psychotherapeutic help and counseling. In this sense, the skillful physician often uses the patient's initial request for drug therapy as a starting point for initiating a psychotherapeutic process. In addition to the short-term symptomatic relief thus attained, a positive placebo effect may often contribute to a general attitude of optimism and confidence on the part of the patient.

## Possible effects of psychotherapy upon pharmacotherapy

Most of the discussion in the literature has focused on possible effects of drug therapy upon psychotherapy. Relatively little attention has been paid to the other side of the process—the impact of psychotherapy upon the patient receiving pharmacotherapy. It is interesting to note how seldom this problem is discussed or even mentioned. Nonetheless, the following potential effects can be identified:

**1) Biochemical replacement effect.** Some pharmacotherapists compare psychotropic drug treatment to the conventional nonpsychiatric use of drugs in medicine, especially endocrine agents like insulin for diabetes. For those who hold this view, correction of the presumed neurophysiological dysfunction or deficiency is the critical factor, and psychotherapy is viewed as unnecessary and irrelevant, or at best, neutral. A variation of this single-factor theory is expressed by some proponents of lithium treatment of mania. The most extreme version is proposed by those who advocate megavitamin therapy for schizophrenia. Those holding such views feel that drugs alone are both necessary and sufficient.

**2) Psychotherapy may be symptomatically disruptive.** Some pharmacotherapists believe that psychotherapy may be deleterious to the pharmacological treatment, since symptoms may be aggravated by excessive probing and uncovering of defenses. Some therapists who have worked with depressives and schizophrenics feel that harm is done the patient by psychotherapeutic intervention, particularly during the acute stage, and that during the early recovery process the patient is best left alone to "heal over" and to reconstitute his defenses.

Here, there is a conflict between those who advocate working through underlying conflicts in psychosis and depression and those who support healing over or sealing over and promoting denial, repression and other defenses. The fear is expressed by many pharmacotherapists that psychotherapy, by uncovering areas of conflict, will raise the titer of tension. Implicit in this debate may be the question of timing: What are the appropriate points in the therapeutic plan at which psychotherapy should be pursued as primarily supportive, and at what points is it appropriate to use uncovering, probing insight techniques?

## Toward a unified view and treatment

The combination of drugs and psychotherapy in psychiatric treatment is widely used but little understood. Ultimately, data from controlled trials will resolve some of the therapeutic issues still in doubt. These issues are especially evident in the treatment of depression, where the alternate therapeutic modalities can be related to relatively specific, although only partially validated, theoretical models such as the neurochemical models which explain and justify drug treatment, and the psychodynamic models which underlie most of the psychotherapeutic methods in current use.

The introduction of animal models in research on depression, using subjects able to develop affectional bonds, offers the strong possibility that unifying theories of depression may yet be developed. For example, Scott et al[14] found that the distress vocalization of puppies separated from their mothers can be markedly reduced, specifically by imipramine, without producing abnormal behavior or adverse physiological side effects. It has also been shown that the morbidity and mortality of wild animals recently captured is significantly reduced by the administration of antidepressants. Studies of the effect of separation-induced depression on the biogenic amine systems of the central and peripheral nervous systems complement the studies showing that conditions psychogenically induced can respond to pharmacotherapy.[14,52] Awareness of such findings, should help to bridge the theoretical distance between psychogenesis and biogenesis.

An admirable start in this direction has been made by Akiskal and McKinney,[53] in a tentative unified hypothesis of depression based on both animal and clinical observations that takes into account the interactions of genetic, chemical, developmental and interpersonal factors which impinge on the diencephalic centers of reinforcement. Cole[54] has recently commented in an editorial that from the psychiatrists' point of view depression is an eminently satisfactory disease because it is quite treatable and is recognized by almost everyone as a real illness demanding treatment. Depression is "satisfactory" also because basic research and clinical trials have given us a better knowledge of its psychopathology and neurobiology than we have for the other major mental illnesses.

Nevertheless, despite our quite substantial information about the psychology and biology of depression, we still lack those integrative concepts needed before pharmacotherapy and psychotherapy can be combined in rational treatment programs which are demonstrably more effective than treatment regimens based on one or the other.

## References

1. G.L. Klerman. "Pharmacological Aspects of Depression," in SEPARATION AND DEPRESSION, J.P. Scott & E.C. Senay, Eds.

AAAS Pub. No. 94 (Washington, D.C.: American Association for the Advancement of Science, 1973), page 69.

2. G. Winokur. "Genetic Aspects of Depression," in SEPARATION AND DEPRESSION, *op. cit.*, page 125.

3. G. Winokur, P.J. Clayton & T. Reich. MANIC-DEPRESSIVE ILLNESS (St. Louis, Mo.: C.V. Mosby, 1969).

4. John Bowlby. ATTACHMENT (New York: Basic Books, 1969).

5. C.M. Heinicke. "Parental Deprivation in Early Childhood," in SEPARATION AND DEPRESSION, *op. cit.*, page 141.

6. T. Beck. DEPRESSION, CAUSE AND TREATMENT (Philadelphia: University of Pennsylvania Press, 1967).

7. J. Mendels. CONCEPTS OF DEPRESSION (New York: J. Wiley & Sons, 1970).

8. E. Bibring. "The Mechanism of Depression," in AFFECTIVE DISORDERS, P. Greenacre, Ed. (New York: International Universities Press, 1953).

9. M. Mendelson. PSYCHOANALYTIC CONCEPTS OF DEPRESSION (Springfield, Ill.: Charles C Thomas, 1960).

10. C.B. Ferster. A Functional Analysis of Depression. *American Psychologist* 857 (1973).

11. F.K. Goodwin & W.E. Bunney. "Psychobiological Aspects of Stress and Affective Illness," in SEPARATION AND DEPRESSION, *op. cit.*

12. W.E. Bunney *et al*. The "Switch Process" in the Manic Depressive Illness, I. A Systematic Study of Sequential Behavioral Changes, *Archives of General Psychiatry* 27 (1972): 295.

13. J.J. Schildkraut. NEUROPHARMACOLOGY AND THE AFFECTIVE DISORDERS (Boston: Little, Brown, 1970).

14. J.P. Scott, J.M. Stewart & V.J. DeGhett, "Separation in infant Dogs," in SEPARATION AND DEPRESSION, *op. cit.*

15. C. Kaufman. "Mother Infant Separation in Monkeys, an experimental model," in SEPARATION AND DEPRESSION, *op. cit.*

16. W.T. McKinney, S.J. Suomi & H.F. Harlow. "New Models of Separation and Depression in Rhesus Monkeys," in SEPARATION AND DEPRESSION, *op. cit.*

17. D.F. Klein & J.M. Davis. DIAGNOSIS AND TREATMENT OF PSYCHIATRIC DISORDERS (Baltimore, Md.: Williams & Wilkins, 1969).

18. B. Davis, B.J. Carroll & R.M. Mowbray. DEPRESSIVE ILLNESS: SOME RESEARCH STUDIES, (Springfield, Ill.: Charles C Thomas, 1972).

19. A.J. Prange. The use of Drugs in Depression: its Theoretical and Practical Basis, *Psychiatric Annals* 3:2 (1973): 56.

20. A.J. Prange, I.C. Wilson, A.E. Knox, T.K. McClane & M.A. Lipton. Enhancement of Imipramine by Thyroid Stimulating Hormone: Clinical and Theoretical Implications, *American Journal of Psychiatry* 127 (1973): 191.

21. A.J. Prange, I.C. Wilson, P.P. Lara & L.B. Alltop. "Effects of Thyrotropin-Releasing Hormone in Depression," in THE THYROID AXIS DRUGS AND BEHAVIOR, A.J. Prange, Ed. (New York: Raven Press, 1974).

22. M. Kac. Some Mathematical Models in Science, *Science* 166 (1969): 695.

23. K. Abraham. "Notes on the Psychoanalytic Investigation and Treatment of Manic-Depressive Insanity and allied Conditions," in SELECTED PAPERS ON PSYCHOANALYSIS (London, England: Hogarth Press, 1927).

24. S. Freud. "Mourning and Melancholia," in STANDARD EDITION, (London, England: Hogarth Press, 1957).

25. E.S. Paykel. "Life Events and Acute Depression" in SEPARATION AND DEPRESSION, *op. cit.*

26. E. Jacobson. THE SELF AND THE OBJECT WORLD (New York: International Universities Press, 1964).

27. E. Weiss. Clinical Aspects of Depression, *Psychoanalytic Quarterly* 13 (1944): 445.

28. M.B. Cohen, G. Baker, R.A. Cohen, F. Fromm-Reichman & E.V. Weigert. An Intensive Study of Twelve Cases of Manic-depressive Psychosis, *Psychiatry* 17 (1954): 103.

29. R.W. Gibson. COMPARISON OF THE FAMILY BACKGROUND AND EARLY LIFE EXPERIENCE OF THE MANIC-DEPRESSIVE AND SCHIZOPHRENIC PATIENT. Final Report, Office of Naval Research Contract Nanr-751 00. (Washington D.C.: Washington School of Psychiatry, 1957).

30. M. Ostow. DRUGS IN PSYCHOANALYSIS AND PSYCHOTHERAPY (New York: Basic Books, 1962).

31. M.S. Sarwer-Foner. THE DYNAMICS OF PSYCHIATRIC DRUG THERAPY (Springfield, Ill.: Charles C Thomas, 1960).

32. H. Azima. Psychodynamic and Psychotherapeutic Problems in Connection with Imipramine (Tofranil) Intake, *Journal of Mental Science* 197 (1961): 74.
33. L. Bellak & S. Rosenberg. Effects of Antidepressant Drugs on Psychodynamics, *Psychosomatics* 7 (1966): 106.
34. G.L. Klerman & E. Gershon. Imipramine Effects Upon Hostility in Depression, *Journal of Nervous Mental Disease* 150 (1970): 12.
35. L.A. Gottschalk, G.C. Gleser, H.W. Wylie & S.M. Kaplan. Effects of Imipramine on Anxiety Hostility Levels, *Psychopharmacologia* 7 (1965): 303.
36. E.J. Sachar. "Endocrine Factors in Psychopathological States," in BIOLOGICAL PSYCHIATRY, J. Mendels, Ed. (New York: J. Wiley & Sons, 1973).
37. E.L. Bliss, V.B. Wilson & J. Zwanziger. Changes in Brain Norepinephrine in Self-Stimulating and "Aversive" Animals, *Journal of Psychiatric Research* 4 (1966): 59.
38. W.E. Bunney, J.D. Mason, J.F. Roatch & D.A. Hamburg. A Psychoendrocrine Study of Severe Psychotic Depressive Crises, *American Journal of Psychiatry* 122 (1965): 72.
39. G.R. Breese, R.D. Smith, R.A. Mueller, J.L. Howard, A.J. Prange & M.A. Lipton. Induction of Adrenal Catecholamine Synthesising Enzymes following Mother-Infant Separation, *Nature New Biology* 246, 151 (1973): 94.
40. E. Lindemann. Symptomatology and Management of Acute Grief, *American Journal of Psychiatry* 101 (1944): 141.
41. A.S. Friedman. The Interaction of Drug Therapy with Marital and Family Therapy in Depressive Patients. Abstract of a paper presented at the 64th Annual Meeting of the American Psychopathological Society, March 7, 1974.
42. L. Covi, R.S. Lipman, L.R. Derogatis, J.E. Smith & J.H. Pattison. Drugs and Group Psychotherapy in Neurotic Depression, *American Journal of Psychiatry* 131, 2 (1974): 191.
43. L. Covi *et al.* Outpatient Treatment of Neurotic Depression. Abstract of a paper presented at the 64th Annual Meeting of the American Psychopathological Society, March 7, 1974.
44. G.L. Klerman, A. DiMascio, M. Weissman, B. Prusoff & E.S. Paykel. Treatment of Depression by Drugs and Psychotherapy, *American Journal of Psychiatry* 131, 2 (1974): 186.

45. T.S. Szasz. Some Observations on the Use of Tranquilizing Drugs, *AMA Archives of Neurology & Psychiatry* 77 (1957): 86.
46. J.A. Meerloo. Medication into Submission: The Danger of Therapeutic Coercion, *Journal of Nervous & Mental Disease* 122 (1955): 353.
47. P.F. Seitz. Experiments in the Substitution of Symptoms by Hypnosis, *Psychosomatic Medicine* 15 (1953): 405.
48. N.E. Miller. Some Recent Studies of Conflict Behavior and Drugs, *American Psychologist* 16 (1961): 12.
49. _____. Some Animal Experiments Pertinent to the Problem of Combining Psychotherapy with Drug Therapy, *Comprehensive Psychiatry* 7 (1966): 1.
50. D. Overton, State-dependent or 'Dissociated' Learning Produced with Pentobarbital, *Journal of Comparative & Physiological Psychology* 57 (1964): 3.
51. A. Wikler. THE RELATION OF PSYCHIATRY TO PHARMACOLOGY (Baltimore, Md.: Williams & Wilkins 1957).
52. W.T. McKinney, L.D. Young, S.J. Suomi & J.M. Davis. Chlorpromazine Treatment of Disturbed Monkeys, *Archives of General Psychiatry* 29 (1973): 490.
53. H.S. Akiskal & W.T. McKinney. Depressive Disorders: Toward a Unified Hypothesis, *Science* 182 (1973): 20.
54. J. Cole. "Depression" (Editorial), *American Journal of Psychiatry* 131 (1974): 204.

# 5

## IMPACT OF PHARMACOTHERAPY ON THE THEORY OF ANXIETY AND THE DYNAMICS OF THE NEUROSES

The relevance of pharmacotherapy to our understanding and treatment of the neuroses has not been marked, but pharmacotherapy has contributed to our understanding of the anxiety or panic attack.

In the anxiety attack the subject is suddenly overwhelmed by fearful sensations accompanied by massive sympathetic and parasympathetic autonomic responses, in particular tachycardia or palpitations, sweating, dizziness, dry mouth, hot and cold flashes, diarrhea, vomiting, sensations of fainting, and fear of death. Although panic anxiety appears indistinguishable from the reaction to overwhelming threat (e.g., being threatened with death), the neurotic anxiety attack is typically characterized by its sudden occurrence without apparent precipitant.

### Psychoanalytic and learning theories of anxiety

The theory of anxiety has gone through three major stages in psychoanalytic thinking. Originally, anxiety was viewed as the direct economic conversion of libido during repression. Later, anxiety was held to be the direct expression of an upsurge of repressed unconscious drives. Still later, anxiety was understood as an affective signal under conditions of anticipated pain or stress. This anticipated distress derived either from the environment or from the breakdown of defenses against repressed drives and affects and the anticipated punishment for their expression. This has become known as signal anxiety. It is evident that the phenomenon of anxiety lends itself to a number of interpretations.

In the neurotic states, the onset of panic anxiety is typically abrupt and does not occur after a long period of mounting anticipatory or signal anxiety. If anything, the exact reverse is true. The signal anxiety develops after the abrupt unheralded onset of the panic attacks. The phobic elaborations are mostly concerned with the subject's attempts to prevent the onset of panic attacks situationally (e.g., refusing to be alone), or to obtain assurance of assistance, through the accessibility of doctors, should he be rendered helpless by panic attack.

For most psychiatrists, the value of discriminating the anxieties and selecting the acute panic attack as worthy of special study is not apparent. Following Freud, anxiety attacks are ordinarily considered simply a quantitative extension of anxiety, without any qualitative uniqueness. Freud distinguishes three forms of neurotic anxiety in Lecture 25 of his INTRODUCTORY LECTURES ON PSYCHOANALYSIS.[1] These are:

> A general apprehensiveness, a kind of freely floating anxiety which is ready to attach itself to any idea that is in any way suitable.... We call this state 'expectant anxiety'.... People who are tormented by this kind of anxiety always foresee the most frighful of all possibilities, interpret every chance event as a premonition of evil and exploit every uncertainty in a bad sense.
>
> A second form of anxiety...is attached to particular objects or situations.... This is the anxiety of the..."phobias."
>
> The third of the forms of neurotic anxiety faces us with the puzzling fact that here the connection between anxiety and a threatening danger is completely lost to view...it may make its appearance, divorced from any determinants and equally incomprehensible to us and to the patient, as an unrelated attack of anxiety.... Yet these conditions...have to be equated with anxiety in all clinical and etiological respects.

Fenichel,[2] in his discussion of anxiety, proposes the hypothesis that the panic attack differs from normal neurotic anxiety only in the sense that panic anxiety occurs when the individual is locked in a tremendous intrapsychic defensive struggle. This struggle, although covert, is of such intensity that the patient is in a situation similar to that of someone lighting a match in a powder factory, so that the signal anxiety is immediately transmuted into panic anxiety.

Learning theory has dealt with the notion of fear and anxiety in a number of ways. Outstanding names in this area are Mowrer,[3] Miller[4] and Tolman.[5] Briefly, Miller views fear as an innate response to painful or noxious stimulation. He views fear also as a response which produces strong stimulation and therefore has impelling or drive property. Miller further views fear as a cue providing information that can function as a generalizing or mediating stimulus. Mowrer is quite close to Tolman, who states that the conditioned stimulus comes to function as a sign of the unconditioned stimulus through the mediation of the fear response, which provides "meaning" to the sign.

The similarity of this formulation to the notion of signal anxiety seems clear. The organism experiences pain and through contiguous experience recognizes those antecedent neutral signs that herald the oncoming painful situation. The organism then develops conditioned "signal" anxiety to the previously neutral stimuli, thus fearfully anticipating the potentially painful situation. Since the fear response is highly activating, one more easily learns the tactics of effective avoidance or mastery behavior.

There has been considerable speculation about other meanings for anxiety in psychotic and borderline states. Some analysts have hypothesized that neuroses may often be defensive against psychotic breaks, so that the therapist must not free the patient from his anxiety defense without prior therapeutically induced structural change in his ego. Regardless of the specific hypothesis about the formation and function of anxiety, there is some agreement in psychoanalytic circles that the symptomatic treatment of anxiety may be either directly harmful to the patient by producing a yet graver disorder or—since anxiety is considered the motor of therapy—harmful to the development of exploratory psychotherapy.

## Pharmacotherapy of panic and anxiety

There has been no attempt as yet to reconcile such formulations with the startling findings accumulated over the past decade concerning the utility of antidepressant agents, in particular imipramine, in blocking anxiety attacks among agoraphobic and school-phobic patients.

One semantic problem is the label "antidepressant" as applied to the two major groups: tricyclics and MAO inhibitors. Labeling a drug in terms of its earliest salient action unfortunately narrows the field of its use. If cortisone had been labeled an antiarthritic, its utility as a hyperglycemic or antiallergic agent would have been obscured. That MAO inhibitors or tricyclics first achieved public acceptance in the treatment of depression should not limit their range of actions. This argument applies also to antipsychotic agents.

The clinical fact, affirmed by double-blind placebo-controlled studies, is that panic attacks are blocked, in almost all cases completely, by the administration of imipramine.[6-9] Some uncontrolled clinical reports[10] indicate similar results with MAO inhibitors. Nonetheless, the anticipatory, signal or expectant anxiety is not immediately affected, although the actual occurrence of panic attacks is relieved. The patient maintains the anxious expectation that a panic attack may occur at any moment and therefore insists on his phobic-dependent maneuvers. It is usually only after a sustained period of being panic-free under medication and supportive-directive psychotherapeutic treatment that he will venture the attempt to abandon his phobic-dependent maneuvers and broaden his horizons.

Drug treatment of the anticipatory anxiety component is possible through the use of sedative agents or minor tranquilizers. With appropriate dosage, patients may expand their constricted horizons more rapidly. In fact, many of these patients have learned that their anticipatory anxiety is allayed by alcohol or barbiturates and run a real risk of becoming addicted. Their panic anxiety, however, is in no way helped by alcohol, barbiturates, or minor tranquilizers.

Although it has been hypothesized that such anxiety represents the threat of incipient psychosis, the use of antipsychotic agents has been conspicuously unsuccessful, usually exacerbating the patient's distress. Further, the occurrence of psychosis in agoraphobics whose symptoms have been successfully treated with antidepressants is very rare. It is therefore unlikely that anticipatory anxiety and panic anxiety represent simply quantitative variants of the same phenomenon. Anticipatory anxiety responds fairly well to minor tranquilizers, sedatives or alcohol but does not respond to antidepressants. Panic anxiety responds to antidepressants but not to minor tranquilizers, sedatives or alcohol. As noted, major tranquilizers usually exacerbate panic anxiety. The therapeutic utility of major tranquilizers in anticipatory anxiety is thus uncertain.

These findings also cast doubt on the theory that psychosis simply represents a further breakdown in the defenses against anxiety. It would be very strange that the antipsychotic agents are effective against the most severe form of mental illness, the psychoses, yet ineffective against lesser forms, if these forms were really only quantitative variations along one dimension rather than qualitatively different illnesses. Clinical anecdotal data suggest that even massive dosage with minor tranquilizers does not prevent psychotic decompensation, thus supporting a clear-cut qualitative distinction between neurotic and psychotic process.

To complete the argument, it should be demonstrable that antipsychotic medication is ineffective against neurotic anxiety. Here the data are contradictory. Some studies affirm the ineffectiveness of antipsychotics, whereas others indicate their effectiveness. One possibility is that states of agitated depression, which may be responsive to antipsychotic medication, are being confused with states of expectant anxiety, which may not be. All these possibilities require careful comparative studies for proper evaluation. In sum, then, we are presented with a group of clinical observations that are at variance with the usual conceptualization of neurotic process in general, agoraphobia in particular, and the relation of neurosis to psychosis. Testing this concept with independent, controlled studies of the antidepressant treatment of school phobia and agoraphobia would be of great heuristic and practical value.

## Psychophysiological aspects of anxiety attacks

Another approach to the anxiety attack is the recent finding by Pitts and McClure[11] that anxiety attacks could be induced in anxiety neurotics by intravenous sodium lactate given under double-blind saline-controlled conditions.

Kelly et al[12] tested this report on 20 patients suffering from anxiety neurosis and 10 normal controls; 16 of the patients experienced an anxiety attack during sodium lactate infusion, as compared with only 1 during normal saline infusion; none of the controls experienced an anxiety attack during saline infusion as compared with 1 during sodium lactate infusion. Provocatively, 8 patients who had experienced lactate-induced anxiety attack were subsequently treated with MAO inhibitor antidepressants. Those who responded well clinically experienced fewer symptoms during a repeat lactate infusion. Among the 5 much-improved patients there were no apparent anxiety attacks. Kelly states,

We were impressed by individual variation of the response to the infusion. Some patients experienced the physiological concomitants of anxiety without the degree of mental fear normally associated with them, while others found that there were only minor discrepancies in symptomatology distinguishing a naturally occurring anxiety attack from the biochemically induced one. Although a number of the controls experienced many symptoms during the infusion, the percentage of anxiety attacks were very much less than in the patient group. This may be because normal controls deal with sodium lactate biochemically in a different way from anxious patients, who have a low threshold for attacks; or alternatively, since anxiety attacks are very rare phenomena in normal people, they require a greater stimulus to precipitate them.

One criticism of the lactate-induced anxiety attack data is that such patients may have been conditioned to respond in an anxious fashion to the peripheral indicators of anxiety. Therefore, it may be that their peripheral psysiology is really not much different from the physiology of the normal person, but they have been so conditioned that they become extremely fearful upon experiencing the peripheral effects of the infusion. The conditioning possibility is rendered somewhat less likely by the prophylactic effect of the MAO inhibitors administered these patients. However, the specificity of MAO-I drugs in this usage is not established, since other drugs have not been tested.

## Attempted integration of clinical data with theory

Studies of adult agoraphobics[6-9] yielded the finding that approximately half of them had manifest early separation anxiety and their illness was precipitated by object loss at an early age. This finding prompted trials of imipramine in school-phobic children, which showed that both clinically and under double-blind placebo-controlled conditions, imipramine blocked panic attacks otherwise occurring in circumstances of attempted separation.

Studies of both adult agoraphobics and school-phobic children emphasize the relationship of panic anxiety to separation anxiety. Nevertheless, approximately half of the adult agoraphobics who respond to imipramine do not have a history of manifest childhood separation anxiety but rather one of late onset that is not obviously precipitated by interpersonal loss and which occurs in some context of rapid endocrine fluctuation caused by hysterectomy, oophorectomy, postpartum state or thyroid disease.

It may be possible to tie together these apparently disparate findings. The hypothesis closely resembles that of John Bowlby[13,14] concerning the development of separation anxiety. Freud proposed a learning theory of separation anxiety, stating that separation anxiety occurs when the infant, prey to mounting instinctual tensions, finds that his discomforts are regularly relieved in the presence of the mothering object but mount in her absence. Separation anxiety then is defined as being due to the anticipation of rising tension and pain under specific learned environmental conditions.

However, observations on animals indicate states of distress after separation from nest or mother in individuals who could not yet have learned that separation means failure to gain relief from instinctual tension. Two examples are the "lost piping" of chicks separated from the nest and the whining of puppies separated from the mother. Both behaviors occur long before any actual drive tension could conceivably have been experienced or before any opportunity to associate maternal absence with endogenous distress. A third example is the separation anxiety which occurs when infant monkeys raised in peer groups are separated from each other. Mothering does not exist in such groups yet separation distress is extreme when an infant is taken from the group.

The members of this Committee hypothesize that separation anxiety may be learned, but learned upon the substrate of an innate biological mechanism. This innate affective control causes intense psychic distress under conditions of naïve separation, with the evolutionary "purpose" of causing the vulnerable infant to emit signals that will elicit retrieval by the mothering parent or by others. Obviously, the helpless dependent infant that has wandered away from the mother is fair game for predators. Further, if the mother cannot find the infant for want of some signal, the infant may well become dehydrated and weakened. If the infant organism waited for the actual hunger pain before emitting retrieval signals, many infants would be lost or impaired. Evolutionarily, a built-in (unlearned) early warning alarm system for the recall of the parent makes good sense.

It is also possible that this alarm system serves as an innate device by which the parent may exert control over the infant at a distance. For instance, ducklings walking to the water with their mother may be instantly recalled when a hawk flies overhead, to huddle under the mother's wings. The mother, perceiving the hawk, emits a distinctive signal that is not used under other circumstances. In this situation, the separation anxiety mechanism serves as a dynamic tie between mother and child, bringing the mother to the child or the child to the mother under appropriate circumstances.

Plainly, any biological control mechanism has a wide range of variations in strength and threshold. It is certainly conceivable that some children have constitutional vulnerabilities in this area that may be exacerbated by maternal practices; and that others may have familial diatheses. The existence of such an innate alarm mechanism may explain the unique specificity of the antidepressants. It is possible that the antidepressants specifically raise the threshold of this mechanism. This would then defuse the panic attack, although the learned anticipatory anxiety developed secondarily to the panic attack would remain unaffected.

If the panic attacks are the cause of the anticipatory anxiety, one would expect that little anticipatory anxiety would develop when only a few panics have occurred. This is the case, as observed in patients successfully treated with imipramine, who relapse on discontinuation of the drug. Regularly, these patients immediately resume the imipramine, which blocks further attacks, and they do not develop anticipatory anxiety or phobic construction of behavior.

This might also offer some explanation for the untoward emergence of panic attacks in persons abruptly deranged endocrinologically. One might speculate that such persons have experienced an artificial lowering of the threshold of the separation anxiety mechanism, resulting in a similar syndrome from a different cause that is restored to normal levels by antidepressants.

It is striking that antidepressant drugs should operate in this fashion, but it is not certain that they all do. Some investigators believe that imipramine is far more effective than either amitryptiline or the MAO inhibitors, but comparative controlled studies to substantiate this have yet to be conducted.

The pathophysiology of separation anxiety and depression are intricately related, as shown by their drug reactivity. This relationship has also frequently been noted in psychodynamic studies. Bowlby points out that the normal response to separation consists of three stages: protest, despair and detachment. The stage of protest appears to be similar to the symptomatolgy of the anxiety attack except for its clear-cut reactive nature, and is also characterized by pleading, clinging and demanding.

More speculatively, the stage of despair may also serve an evolutionary purpose. If an infant is separated from its mother the correct pro-survival behavior would seem to be to make a fuss and thus elicit retrieval. If retrieval is not effected in fairly short order, the mothering figure may be incapacitated, at least temporarily. Therefore, continued protest would only serve as an antisurvival function by attracting predator notice and exhausting infant energy reserves. Thus, the state of despair may well serve as a built-in conservation mechanism. It is conceivable that separation anxiety and depression both stem from an impairment in the evolved control mechanisms which deal with the evolutionarily crucial situation of emergency separation.

One might speculate still further about the stage of detachment. Here too an evolutionary function is possible, since the "detached" child would then be able to turn toward new objects with relative ease and accept them as foster parents. Evolution may thus have been molded by the experience of fostering among social animals. If the tie to the mother were to remain unbreakable, the despairing infant could not respond to the foster mother. Therefore, a mechanism for detachment becomes biologically necessary to all fostering.

Since psychopathy—characterized by the inability to attach emotionally to others, identify with them, and care for them—has been reported as a complication of marked object deprivation during early fostering, it is conceivable that cryptogenic psychopathy may be secondary to derangements of the hypothesized detachment mechanism.

To sum up, the new clinical observations derived from the effects of antidepressants, minor tranquilizers and major tranquilizers on anxiety attacks provide material that calls for modification of existing dynamic theory in many crucial theoretical areas.

### References

1. S. Freud. "Introductory Lectures on Psychoanalysis," in STANDARD EDITION (London, England: Hogarth Press, 1963), Vol. XVI, quoted by permission of the publisher.
2. O. Fenichel. PSYCHOANALYTIC THEORY OF NEUROSIS (New York: W.W. Norton, 1945).

3. O.H. Mowrer. Two Factor Learning Theory: Summary and Comment, *Psychology Review* 58 (1951): 350.

4. N.E. Miller. "Learnable Drives and Rewards," in HANDBOOK OF EXPERIMENTAL PSYCHOLOGY, S.S. Stevens, Ed. (New York: John Wiley & Sons, 1951).

5. E.C. Tolman. PURPOSIVE BEHAVIOR IN ANIMALS AND MEN (New York: Appleton-Century-Crofts, 1932).

6. D.F. Klein. Delineation of Two Drug-Response Anxiety Syndromes, *Psychopharmacologia* 5 (1964): 397.

7. _____. Importance of Psychiatric Diagnosis in Prediction of Clinical Drug Effects, *Archives of General Psychiatry* 16 (1967): 118.

8. R. Gittelman-Klein & D.F. Klein. Controlled Imipramine Treatment of School Phobia, *Archives of General Psychiatry* 25 (1971): 204.

9. _____. "School Phobia. Diagnostic Considerations in the Light of Imipramine Effects," in DRUGS, DEVELOPMENT AND CEREBRAL FUNCTION, L. Smith, Ed. (Springfield, Ill.: Charles C Thomas, 1972).

10. D. Kelly, W. Guirguis, E. Frommer, N. Mitchell-Heggs & W. Sargent. Treatment of Phobic States with Antidepressants, *British Journal of Psychiatry* 116 (1970): 387.

11. F.N. Pitts & J.N. McClure. Lactate Metabolism in Anxiety Neurosis, *New England Journal of Medicine* 277 (1967): 1329.

12. D. Kelly, N. Mitchell-Heggs & D. Sherman. Anxiety and the Effects of Sodium Lactate Assessed Clinically and Physiologically, *British Journal of Psychiatry* 119 (1971): 129.

13. J. Bowlby. Separation Anxiety, *International Journal of Psychoanalysis* 41 (1960): 89.

14. _____. ATTACHMENT (New York: Basic Books, 1969).

# 6

## DRUGS AND PSYCHOANALYSIS

Psychoanalysis is deeply rooted in biology and was derived from the neurobiology of the 19th century. No one recognized better than Freud the limitations of psychoanalysis as a therapeutic tool. With an appropriate synthesis of his biological background and his clinical concern for the patient's welfare, he wrote in his posthumously published OUTLINE OF PSYCHOANALYSIS:[1]

> The future may teach us how to exercise a direct influence, by means of particular chemical substances, upon the amounts of energy and their distribution in the apparatus of the mind. It may be that there are other undreamed-of possibilities of therapy. But for the moment we have nothing better at our disposal than the technique of psychoanalysis, and for that reason, in spite of its limitations, it is not to be despised.

As early as 1928 he had said:

> Because of the essential unity of the two things that we divide into somatic and psychic, one may prophesy that the day will come when the avenue from biology and chemistry to the phenomenon of neurosis will be open for our understanding and we hope also for therapy.[2]

What were the limitations to psychoanalysis of which Freud spoke? Paraphrasing his conclusions reached in "Analysis Terminable and Interminable."[3] Anna Freud[4] writes that in Freud's view the primary limitations were the quantitative ones which determine the libido economy within a given individual and are decisive for his inner equilibrium, i.e., for the balance or imbalance in the defensive struggle between id and ego. Any excessive strength of instinct whether constitutionally given or due to developmental reinforcement (puberty, menopause) may make it more difficult or impossible for analysis to achieve its main task, i.e., to tame the instincts. Any weakening of the ego, whether through illness or exhaustion, or from some similar cause may have the same effect.

These difficulties, as pointed out by Strachey[5] are of a physiological and biological nature and thus in the main considered not susceptible to psychological influences.

In the same essay Freud[3] described other difficulties which he considered to be qualitative in nature. Alterations of the ego, "whether original or innate" or "acquired during the earliest defensive struggles of the earliest years," which have limited the plasticity and versatility of the defenses, that is, "physical inertia," are a great source of difficulty, often making the personality of even very young patients "fixed and rigid."

Other difficulties he attributed to the results of "flooding" by distressing id material when defenses have been reduced; this could lead to negative therapeutic reactions. Still others in his view depend upon elements of free aggression which, when turned inward, produce "an ominous alteration from the search for pleasure as a governing principle to the preference for unpleasure."

Adding to the difficulties recognized in 1937, Anna Freud[4] later suggests others: (1) "a low threshold of tolerance for the frustration of instinctual wishes," (2) "a low threshold of tolerance for anxiety," (3) "a low sublimation potential," and (4) "a preponderance of regressive over progressive tendencies." She proposes as remedies alterations in psychoanalytic emphasis, such as the interpretation of defenses before id impulses, and the so-called analysis of the total personality. She also discusses the possibility of analysis of the first year of life. She cogently questions the assumption that whatever is acquired early in life is irreversible, emphasizing that this is not proved. In monkeys at least, where serious behavior disturbances can be generated by early life experiences, McKinney *et al* have shown that disturbances can be reversed by "monkey therapists" or by chlorpromazine.[6]

There can be little doubt that Freud, who had early experience with the dramatic mood-altering properties of cocaine, must have been fully aware of the potential of psychotropic drugs. However, prior to 1940 the drugs available were limited in both potency and specificity. Nonetheless, interest in the biological bases of drives and their interaction with defenses is not new among psychoanalysts. The monograph by Benedek and Rubinstein[7] demonstrating alterations in the intensity and duration of sexual impulses and defenses against them in women at different stages of their menstrual cycle is a classic of feasibility and methodological rigor in psychoanalytic investigation of biological influence.

It is easy enough to understand why prior to 1940, when drugs were relatively unpotent, Freud defended the psychoanalytic technique as something "not to be despised" despite its limitations. But in principle the revolution in psychopharmacological drugs since the early 1950's should have altered the situation considerably. Moreover, advances in biology have shown that the expression of the hereditary endowment of man is not fixed and immutable. Genotypes need not necessarily express themselves as specific and unalterable phenotypes. In illustration, many psychotropic drugs certainly diminish anxiety, perhaps by their influence on the intensity of instinctual drives. Presumably when appropriately utilized they should alter response and prepare the organism for optimal psychoanalytic therapy.

One might have predicted that psychoanalysts would have

welcomed Freud's projections into the future and would have taken them seriously. Instead, many have warned against drugs as impediments to therapy; have denied their utility; have barred them from discussion in the psychoanalytic journals. Most seriously, and with few exceptions, they have ignored the opportunities for systematic research into the mode of action of the various new drugs on the psychic apparatus in metapsychological terms, and into possibilities for extending their range of applicability in practice and theory to broader case material. Why there should be such resistance is a matter of speculation.

Because the therapeutic model in psychoanalysis is the development of the transference neurosis and its working through, analysts have invariably resisted the introduction of noninterpretive techniques. Thus, they have generally resisted what in the psychoanalytic literature are called "parameters," which involve such measures as advice (even medical advice), direction, gratification of dependency needs, and role-playing.[8] They have also tended to resist intrusions upon the strict privacy of the analytic interview such as tape recordings or use of the one-way screen. It is understandable, then, that they should resist the use of drugs, assuming that the transaction of administering anything from a physical examination to a drug will in itself distort or contaminate the transference. Drugs in particular have been endowed by some analysts with almost magical properties. It is also assumed by some that drugs will impede therapy by fostering regression, reducing anxiety, and especially by offering sufficient symptomatic relief to induce the patient to discontinue therapy. It is because of all these reservations that some analysts state with apparent pride that they have never prescribed drugs.

Such fears do not seem realistic in light of the facts. Drugs can be administered in such a way as to exclude the factor of "magic." Their effectiveness in fostering regression and eliminating anxiety is far from absolute and can be controlled by dosage adjustment or even discontinuation. There is no evidence in the contemporary literature that drugs actually impede therapy.

None of this is meant to imply that drugs should be employed in all psychoanalytic psychotherapy. Quite the contrary, for many patients do not require them. Some require them only in very specific tactical situations, while for others they may play a major part in the therapeutic strategy. In a few cases drugs may be contraindicated or may cause paradoxical reactions. But a flat and unequivocal denial of their utility is not reasonable and appears to be a resistance rather than an opinion based on evidence.

Compared to the reception of drugs in schizophrenia fifteen years ago, which was highly critical, the treatment of schizophrenia today without drugs is almost unthinkable. Anna Freud[4] says,

> Analysts have to admit that where quantitatively massive upheavals of the personality are concerned, such as in the psychoses, the purely psychological methods by themselves are inadequate and the organic and chemical means have the advantage over them. They do not concede the same for the neuroses.

Comparing psychoanalysis with other psychotherapies she says,

> In competition with the psychotherapies they [psychoanalysts] are justified to maintain that what they have to offer is unique, i.e., thoroughgoing personality changes as compared with more superficial symptomatic cures. Unfortunately, the former is not always aspired to by the patients who aim above all at immediate relief from suffering.

It is the more regrettable that so little research goes on in this

area. Nonetheless, from what has been done it seems safe to
hypothesize the following:

1.  The use of psychopharmacologic drugs permits psycho-
    analytic treatment of a broader spectrum of patients than
    would otherwise be amenable to such treatment. These
    include psychoneurotics, depressives, pseudoneurotic
    schizophrenics, potential schizophrenics, and other types
    of acting-out patients.
2.  Hospitalization can by this means frequently be avoided in
    the management of these patients.
3.  Psychoactive drugs may facilitate the psychoanalytic proc-
    ess when it has bogged down.
4.  There is no reported evidence that appropriate drug use
    alters or impedes the process of psychoanalytic psycho-
    therapy.

## Psychoanalytic research with drugs

Fortunately, a few psychoanalysts have been concerned with
the role of drugs in psychoanalysis and psychoanalytic
therapy and over the years have published data and conclusions relevant not only to the utility of drugs but also to their
modes of interaction. Ostow,[9-12] for example, has from his
extensive experience with such agents formulated the theory,
based upon Freud's libido theory, that tranquilizers and antidepressants affect mental illness by influencing the "libidinal
energy available to the ego for drive discharge." He theorizes
that tranquilizers diminish the ego supply of libido, whereas
energizers increase supply. Accordingly, Ostow employs
drugs during the course of psychoanalysis to control "available psychic energy" in order to reinforce the stabilizing effect
of the analysis itself or to attenuate the possible disruptive
effect of the transference neurosis, or both. He sees drugs and
psychoanalysis to be complementary in that "psychoanalytic
technique alone cannot undo extreme deviations of the ego-
libido supply."[11]

On the other hand, Ostow believes that psychopharmacological agents alone can neither achieve the effect of proper
psychoanalytic interpretations, nor substitute for them, nor
can drug therapy alone improve family relations, love relations, self-esteem or similar phenomena which give rise to
neurotic or psychotic illness. Ostow claims that combinations
of psychoanalytic technique and psychoactive drug therapy
offer him a much greater degree of control of the patient's
symptoms and behavior than can be achieved by either alone.
Although techniques are difficult to work out because of the
problem of finding the precise drug dosages in the individual
case, he reports good results in difficult patients with combined therapy. However, systematic clinical tabulations are
not presented in his reports.

Gottschalk has obtained objective data which may lend
some support to Ostow's libido or psychic-energy theory of
psychoactive drug effects. Specifically, a drug-placebo
double-blind cross-over study of the effects of perphenazine
on the content of verbal behavior revealed a significant decrease in the outward level of hostility in the speech of
patients,[13] whereas in another study[14] imipramine as compared to a placebo increased hostility outward. Although
libidinal energy and aggressive energy are not necessarily
related, Ostow's concepts would be supported by this work if
outward-directed hostility may be considered inferential evidence of levels of psychic energy.

Ostow's psychic-energy model for the mode of action of the
various psychoactive drugs is a first approximation, and in
some instances his theoretical postulations are controverted
by clinical experience. Ostow's model predicts that
phenothiazines should worsen depression, whereas in actual
clinical usage they have often proved highly useful. Nonetheless, he is one of the few psychoanalytic investigators who has
even attempted a systematic formulation of psychoactive drug
action in metapsychological terms and who has reported on
his experience of orthodox psychoanalytic treatment proce-

dures combined with virtually all the currently available psychoactive agents.[12]

Sarwer-Foner[15] was another of the early psychoanalytic investigators to study psychodynamic effects of psychoactive drugs. In contrast to Ostow's, Azima's, and Winkleman's explanations of the actions of psychoactive drugs—which focus on instinct, drive and instinctual energy and which assume that reintegrative changes in the personality result from drug induced alterations in these drives or energetics—Sarwer-Foner focuses on ego defenses. To him, inner drives are not necessarily directly influenced by psychoactive drugs, but their expression is altered in the activity level of the patient's musculoskeletal system or other physical aspects of relating himself to the world. The ability to translate these drives into action is controlled or partially controlled by the drug.

Since Sarwer-Foner focuses on ego defenses and on the effect of pharmacological agents on coping mechanisms, the experienced effect or "psychological meaning" to the individual patient of the pharmacological action of the drug becomes extremely important. For example, in the case of a highly active patient who uses activity to assure himself that he is not feminine, reduction of overactivity may increase rather than reduce anxiety and agitation. Many other paradoxical reactions are explained by Sarwer-Foner in this fashion. He is particularly concerned about the therapeutic milieu and the patient-physician relationship, commenting as follows:

> The patient who therefore benefits from the characteristic pharmacological profile of the neuroleptic medication does so because he interprets the action of the drug in controlling certain symptoms or symptom complexes as a "good" or "bad." Some of these include the attitude of the doctors, nurses, and orderlies both toward the particular drug and the patient's reaction to receiving it.[15]

Azima and Sarwer-Foner[16] and Bellak (cf. Bellak and

Chassan[17]) have been the only psychoanalysts to employ double-blind controls in obtaining their data. In the 1961 study by Sarwer-Foner and Azima, 4 patients in psychoanalytic psychotherapy were given a series of drugs— chlorpromazine, reserpine, imipramine and two placebos (one inert and the other phenobarbital) over a 2 year period. The drug dose was increased to the level of tolerance and was given over an average of 10 sessions, with 10 medication-free sessions between each drug regimen. The therapists undertook the analytic treatment in a routine manner. They reported that in no case was the therapeutic process accelerated, decelerated, or altered during the periods of drug dosage. Typical pharmacological effects of the drugs were noted when the dosage reached a certain level. The number of remembered dreams increased during the periods of reserpine dosage. Bellak and Chassan[17] employed a longitudinal design in a single case to evaluate the influence of psychoactive drugs (in this study, chlordiazepoxide) in combination with psychoanalytic psychotherapy and reported significant positive effects during the on-drug periods for a variety of ego-function factors. In a more recent study, Bellak et al[18] found similar results for diazepam, also using intensive design and a single patient. The patient showed overall improvement over time as well as specific improvement in various ego-function factors, and the authors state: "The global ego function averages thus obtained show a clear significant difference between diazepam and placebo...."

Still other workers (e.g., Lesse[19]) have reported the use of psychoactive drugs in the treatment of patients either by psychoanalysis or by psychoanalytically oriented therapy. Indeed, it seems highly likely, as indicated by the findings of Hayman,[20] that the use of psychoactive drugs, especially the minor tranquilizers, although infrequently reported, is a more common practice among analysts than they are prepared to acknowledge. In any case, it is regrettable that so few of the studies that are reported use double-blind techniques.

Although it is argued[21,22] that the use of double-blind techniques is antithetical to the clinical concerns of the therapist and to the nature of the therapist-patient contract, it is nonetheless essential to the research value of such work. The capacity for self-deception in open experiments of this type is altogether too well-known. The concept of psychic energy, for example, should be readily testable in double-blind experiments, since Ostow employs scales of libido-energy around which to adjust his dosage. It would be invaluable if he could measure ego-libido and its changes in placebo controlled studies and without knowing the nature or quantity of the drugs employed. Such experiments would be of great theoretical value and need not be inimical to the patients' interests. Many other psychoanalytic concepts could be tested in this way and valuable bridges between drug or hormone-induced biological changes and their metapsychological consequences might be established.

## References

1. Sigmund Freud. AN OUTLINE OF PSYCHOANALYSIS (New York: W.W. Norton, 1949).
2. S. Cobb. BORDERLINES OF PSYCHIATRY (Cambridge, Mass.: Harvard University Press, 1943), Page 127.
3. Sigmund Freud. "Analysis Terminable and Interminable," in STANDARD EDITION (London, England: Hogarth Press, 1937), Vol. 23, pp. 209-253.
4. Anna Freud. DIFFICULTIES IN THE PATH OF PSYCHOANALYSIS (New York: International Universities Press, 1969).
5. John Strachey. "Editor's Note," in Freud's STANDARD EDITION (London, England: Hogarth Press, 1964) Vol. 23, page 211.
6. W.T. McKinney, L.D. Young, S.J. Suomi & J.M. Davis. Chlorpromazine Treatment of Disturbed Monkeys, Archives of General Psychiatry 29 (1973): 490.
7. Therese Benedek & B.B. Rubenstein. "The Sexual Cycle in Women" in PSYCHOSEXUAL FUNCTIONS IN WOMEN, T. Benedek,

Ed. (New York: Ronald Press, 1942) Chapters 1-11. Reprinted in 1952.

8. Franz Alexander. PSYCHOANALYSIS AND PSYCHOTHERAPY (New York: W.W. Norton, 1956).

9. M. Ostow. DRUGS IN PSYCHOANALYSIS AND PSYCHOTHERAPY (New York: Basic Books, 1962).

10. _____. The Struggle against Depression, *Canadian Psychiatric Association Journal* (Suppl. 2 (1966): 5139.

11. _____. "The Complementary Roles of Psychoanalysis and Drug Therapy," in PSYCHIATRIC DRUGS, P. Solomon, Ed., (New York: Grune & Stratton, 1966).

12. _____. "Continuing Drug Needs in Mental Illness and Its Pathogenetic Use." Paper presented at a symposium of the American Psychiatric Association, 1966.

13. L.A. Gottschalk, G.C. Gleser, K.J. Springer, S.M. Kaplan, J. Shanon & W.D. Ross. Effects of Perphenazine on Verbal Behavior Patterns, *AMA Archives of General Psychiatry* 2 (1960): 632.

14. L.A. Gottschalk, G.C. Gleser, H.W. Wylie & S.M. Kaplan. Effects of Imipramine on Anxiety and Hostility Levels Derived from Verbal Communications, *Psychopharmacologia* 7 (1965): 303.

15. G.J. Sarwer-Foner. The Role of Neuroleptic Medication in Psychotherapeutic Interaction, *Comprehensive Psychiatry* 1 (1960): 291.

16. H. Azima & G.J. Sarwer-Foner. Psychoanalytic Formulations of the Effects of Drugs in Pharmacotherapy, *Revue Canadienne de Biologie* 20 (1961): 603.

17. L. Bellak & J.B. Chassan. An Approach to the Evaluation of Drug Effect During Psychotherapy: A Double-blind Study of a Single Case, *Journal of Nervous and Mental Disease* 139 (1964): 20.

18. L. Bellak, J.B. Chassan, H. Gediman *et al.* Ego Function Assessment of Analytic Psychotherapy Combined with Drug Therapy, *Journal of Nervous & Mental Disease* 157 (Dec. 1973): 465-469, at page 467.

19. S. Lesse. Combined Drug and Psychotherapy of Severely Depressed Ambulatory Patients, *Canadian Psychiatric Association Journal* 11 (1966): 5123.

20. M. Hayman. Drugs and the Psychoanalyst, *American Journal of Psychotherapy* 21 (1967): 644.

21. M. Ostow. Method and Madness: A Critique of Current Methodology in Psychiatric Drug Research, *Journal of New Drugs* 5, (1965) 3.
22. _____. Economy in Treatment and Economy in Research, *International Journal of Psychiatry* 8 (1969: 744.

# 7

## THE USE OF DRUGS IN BEHAVIOR THERAPY

### The nature of behavior therapy

Behavior therapy is a growing competitor of psychoanalysis and psychoanalytically oriented or "dynamic" psychotherapy. As a relative newcomer to the field of psychiatry which is evolving rapidly and acquiring its own eclecticism, it merits brief historical review of its theoretical basis, practice, and claims for therapeutic efficacy.

Behavior therapy is based upon theories of learning and conditioning developed by experimental psychologists. Its proponents claim that it is the only psychotherapeutic technique grounded in an established body of theory and empirical evidence that may be considered sound in terms of accepted canons of legitimate scientific methodology. Its more extreme advocates consider behavior therapy competitive with and even antithetical to psychoanalysis and dynamically oriented psychotherapy. The schism between these two schools of psychotherapeutic method has at times been marked by deep and passionate differences. Thus, Eysenck,[1] speaking against orthodox psychoanalysis, says

> The whole story of psychoanalysis is little but a repetition of the famous fairy-tale about the Emperor's new clothes. And it is curious to note that these dissenters tend to be found mostly among those who have been trained in scientific method and who have adopted psychology as their profession. There are very few experimental psychologists or leading psychological theoreticians who accept Freudian doctrine, and the majority tend to regard it as so much beyond

119

the pale that they do not even consider it necessary to discuss and argue its pretensions. We thus have the curious position that psychoanalysis is widely accepted among lay people and others untrained in psychology, ignorant of experimental methods and incapable of evaluating empirical evidence. On the other hand, we have a widespread rejection of psychoanalytic claims by those knowledgeable in psychology, experienced in experimental methodology and well able to evaluate empirical findings. The most obvious hypothesis suggested by this state of affairs would seem to be that psychoanalysis is a myth; a set of semi-religious beliefs disseminated by a group of people who should be regarded as prophets rather than scientists.

Later in the same paper Eysenck gives a succinct formulation of his conception of the principles of behavior therapy:

...no scientific theory has ever been killed by the criticism directed at its inadequacies; what is required is an alternative and clearly superior theory. Such a theory, in my view, is at the moment in the process of being formulated by a number of American and British writers; its theoretical background lies in Pavlovian conditioning and modern learning theory, while its practical application has been labelled "behavior therapy," to indicate its relationship to the tenets of behaviorism. What is maintained by this theory may be put very briefly thus. Neurotic symptoms are maladaptive actions and/or emotions which have become conditioned to certain types of stimuli. They can be removed by an appropriate process of extinction and counter-conditioning. There is no disease underlying these symptoms, and there are no complexes which produce the new symptoms should the old ones be extinguished. All that we are dealing with in a neurosis is, in fact, the symptom or set of symptoms; once they are eliminated, the neurosis, as such, has vanished.

Speaking of the therapeutic effectiveness of conventional psychotherapy and behavior therapy, Eysenck[2] states:

> ...behavior therapy is an alternative type of treatment to psychotherapy; it is a superior type of treatment.... Insofar as psychotherapy is at all effective it is so in virture of certain principles which can be derived from learning theory.... Psychotherapy can be considered a minor part of behavior therapy.

As might be expected, the psychoanalytic rejoinder has sometimes been no less vitriolic. Thus Szasz[3] states:

> They are not competitive therapeutic methods whose relative value is a matter of medical judgment. Instead, the difference between them is more like the difference between an open and closed society. Behavior therapy and psychoanalysis are essentially two rival systems of belief— one full of order, simplicity, and oppression; the other of diversity, complexity , and freedom...whose relative values are a matter of moral judgment.

## New techniques of behavior therapy

In the early phases of developing theory and method, the proponents of behavior therapy were quite dogmatic regarding the strict and exclusive adherence to the principles of learning theory alone. The early work of Jules Masserman,[4] Dollard and Miller[5] and others led to the formulation and development of new techniques by Eysenck, Wolpe, Lazarus, Bandura, and Rachman. Some examples may be noted.

**1. Counter-conditioning, or aversion therapy.** The patient—for example a male homosexual—is administered a painful electric shock upon presentation of a projected image of a nude male.[6,7] Or an alcoholic patient is administered a powerful nausea-producing drug in combination with a favored alcoholic beverage.[8]

**2. Systematic desensitization.** Stimuli of increasing anxiety-provoking intensity for the patient are presented in an order based on his tolerance of each step *without* concurrent anxiety, until the critical problem area is reached and it, too, can be confronted without anxiety. This procedure was originally conducted utilizing the "progressive relaxation" method devised by Jacobson.[9] However, it was soon discovered that this method was ineffective in completely allaying the severe anxiety of many patients and other adjuvants have been used, among them hypnosis, and, as will be discussed later, various psychopharmacological agents. The method of systematic desensitization, in this case utilizing hypnosis, is succinctly described by Bandura[10]:

> On the basis of historical information, interview data and psychological test responses, the therapist constructs a hierarchy, a ranked list of stimuli to which the patient reacts with anxiety. In the case of desensitization based on relaxation, the patient is hypnotized, and is given relaxation suggestions. He is then asked to imagine a scene representing the weakest item on the anxiety hierarchy and, if the relaxation is unimpaired, this is followed by having the patient imagine the next item on the list, and so on. Thus, the anxiety cues are gradually increased from session to session, until the last phobic stimulus can be presented without impairing the relaxed state. Through this procedure, relaxation responses eventually come to be attached to the anxiety-provoking stimuli.

Wolpe[7] has developed a theoretical explanation for this procedure which he calls "reciprocal inhibition." It suggests that the gradual extinction of the anxiety response during desensitization is brought about by repeated pairing with incompatible "relaxation responses."

**3. Operant conditioning** is another technique utilized by behavior therapists. In this method, reward situations are set up to provide positive reinforcement contingent upon the behavior patterns that the therapist hopes to shape and maintain. An example of operant technique is reported in the work of Burchard and Tyler,[11] who achieved a marked decrease in the "destructive and disruptive behavior" of a 13-year-old delinquent boy by systematically isolating him when he behaved in an antisocial way and by rewarding him for socially acceptable behavior.

The token economy (Allyon and Azrin[12]) is based on the operant technique. Here, the desired behavior on the institutional ward is shaped and maintained with reward-associated "tokens" and the undesired behavior is extinguished by withholding tokens.

**4. Assertive training.** This technique is typically carried out[8] by strongly encouraging the patient with maladaptive anxiety responses in interpersonal contexts to "stand up for himself" more. He learns to do so, gradually increasing his capacity to say and do what he thinks reasonable and right by actual performance in concrete life situations. For the patient who has extreme difficulty in initiating such behavior, Wolpe suggests the technique of "behavioral rehearsal" (of psychodrama), which may better prepare the patient for real-life confrontations. Indeed, Wolpe claims that "a good deal of deconditioning of anxiety frequently takes place during the behavior rehearsal itself." It should be noted, however, that he judiciously adds the admonition, "Never instigate an assertive act that is likely to have seriously punishing consequences for the patient."

## Claims of the behaviorists

The claims of behavior therapists for the effectiveness of their procedures may be extravagant in terms of outcome. Indeed, many experienced clinicians only too familiar with the persistent intractability of many neurotic conditions and the somewhat embarrassing rate of relapse and later return to psychotherapy may with justifiable skepticism view these outcome claims as entirely too sanguine. One plausible suspicion that immediately comes to mind concerns that of *patient selection*; another is the *adequacy of the criteria for cure* and/or improvement.

Wolpe[8] unequivocally states that "89% of 210 patients had either apparently recovered or were at least 80% improved in a mean of about 30 therapeutic sessions.... *No case diagnosed as neurotic was refused treatment if time was available.*" [Italics added.] Rachman,[13] while admitting the inadequacy of follow-up studies, claims immediate outcome cure rates approaching 90% for phobic and anxiety states, and Lazarus[14] reports that in his clinical work, of a sample of 126 individuals diagnosed as "extremely neurotic," 61.9% were rated as "markedly improved" or "completely recovered" in a mean of 14.07 sessions; of 408 less severely ill patients, 78% "appeared to derive definitie and constructive benefit." Furthermore, in follow-up studies with a mean duration of 2.15 years, only one patient was considered to have "relapsed," and Lazarus goes on to say that "there was no evidence of relapse in any of the other cases. On the contrary, they appeared not only to have maintained their gains, but in certain instances, to have progressed beyond them."

**Outcome criteria.** As to the question of outcome criteria, Lazarus proffers the following four clinical assessments:

1) Does the patient appear to be completely free from symptoms?
2) Is there evidence that the patient is able to enter into and maintain congenial interpersonal relationships?
3) Can the patient gratify his basic needs and strivings creatively and realistically?

4) Has the patient the facility to endure a certain amount of frustration and deprivation, and the ability to adjust to inimical conditions?

Whatever limitations and/or inadequacies this formulation of successful therapeutic outcome may have in the opinion of some, they certainly cannot claim that it is totally wide of the mark. And if the statistical data for outcome efficacy are to be taken at all seriously as indicative of real therapeutic improvement, the openminded clinician genuinely concerned with finding and utilizing an optimally effective methodology must ask why.

Any conclusive answer to this question will doubtless have to await data from further clinical and experimental research. Whether or not behavior techniques ultimately prove to be as efficacious in widespread clinical usage as their proponents now claim, and whether or not their success, once demonstrated, should prove attributable to the strictly construed principles of learning theory on which they are based, one fact must be noted: In the development of applied behavior therapy over the last decade, most of its leading practitioners have become increasingly eclectic and pragmatic in their actual clinical practice.[15]

**Broad-spectrum vs. strict behavior.** In Wolpe's most recent book,[8] he describes the utilization of a considerable number of techniques that are standard in current clinical psychotherapeutic practice. These include supportive methods, analysis and evaluation of problematic complex interpersonal situations, and even directive measures based on mutual realistic cognitive appraisal of the patient's problem areas.

In a 1969 paper,[16] Lazarus claims that his method, which he calls "broad-spectrum behavior therapy," is often more efficacious than "strict" behavior therapy:

...the routine application of relaxation training, desensitization, aversion-relief and so forth, is extremely tedious and laborious. Futher, these procedures alone are often therapeutically insufficient. Many cases require didactic intervention and emotional reeducation over and above specific conditioning procedures. In addition to (and often in place of) laboratory-derived techniques like systematic desensitization, I tend to focus considerable attention on relationship variables; the patient's system of values, attitudes and beliefs; aspects of high and low self-esteem; practical considerations such as leisure and recreational pursuits; dyadic transactions; and various group processes. One may practice this "technical electicism" within a learning theory framework, but one's allegiance to laboratory studies and laboratory procedures may become extremely tenuous when attempting to decrease the vagaries of emotional suffering, as opposed to eliminating avoidance responses evoked by harmless snakes and spiders. I must plead guilty to the charge of having functioned as a clinician who employed broad-spectrum behavior therapy, and then attributed his results solely to strict behavior therapy (see, for example, Lazarus[14]).

Another therapist reporting successful utilization of combined behavioral and dynamic approaches is Brady.[17] In this paper, Brady suggests that the actual methodology of at least some of the successes with behavior therapy are in fact "more empirical in nature although they too are often rationalized in learning theory terms," and goes on to say:

> ...many authors hold that psychological theories which underlie the two approaches are not mutually exclusive but rather different levels of conceptualization and analysis of the same phenomena. Apropos of this view are efforts to reexamine concepts and principles of psychoanalytic theory and practice from the viewpoint of learning theory. Concepts such as displacement, repression and insight which are central to dynamic theory have been meaningfully analyzed

in conditioning terms. The purpose of such reformulations has not been to replace one terminology or frame of reference with another. Rather, the object has been to gain new perspectives on psychotherapeutic phenomena which may help clarify important theoretical issues and suggest innovations in treatment which are amenable to clinical investigation.

## Behavior therapy and pharmacotherapy

Many advocates of behavior therapy—principally those trained in the nonmedical psychotherapeutic professions— have been more or less resistant to combining psychopharmacological therapy with behavior therapy, although several prominent behavior therapists have adopted pharmacological agents as valuable complements to behavior methods. For example, Wolpe[8] has the following to say:

> ...the use of drugs is never inimical to the achievement of the fundamental changes at which behavior therapy aims; and there is little doubt that in some cases they actively promote such changes. The hazard of addiction is small when the duration of drug treatment is limited. Usually as the neurotic reactions are deconditioned, the dose required for symptomatic relief becomes less, so that it is often possible to discontinue medication altogether a good while before the conclusion of therapy.

Brady[18] also sees great promise in the combination of pharmacotherapy and behavior therapy. Nevertheless, there is a remarkable paucity of work reported and most of what is reported is impressionistic and anecdotal. Virtually no controlled double-blind studies with adequate rating scales, appropriate numbers of cases, and appropriate statistical analyses have appeared in the literature. Yet psychiatrically trained behavior therapists have in fact frequently availed themselves of the entire pharmacological armamentarium.

Wolpe[8] reports using meprobamate (400-800 mg. qid), chlordiazepoxide (10-30 mg. tid) and one or another of the amphetamine-barbiturate combinations (bid). He also reports the use of more potent psychoactive drugs such as various phenothiazine derivatives, MAO inhibitors, and the tricyclic antidepressants, mentioning, in addition, the use of progesterone, testosterone and codeine. As to choice of agent he states, "As every experienced clinician knows, it is trial and error that ultimately decides which drug will be effective in an individual case."[8]

In clinical use, behavior therapists employ drugs in at least four distinct paradigms: (1) as noxious stimuli, (2) as therapeutic adjuvants, (3) for general anxiety reduction, and (4) for immediate and long-range relief of specific target symptoms.

**1. Noxious stimuli.** Drugs such as apomorphine, emetine and ipecac were perhaps among the first pharmacologic agents to be used in behavior therapy.[19,20] They are administered to induce states of nausea and vomiting in patients undergoing aversion training, and have been used for treatment of sexual disorders as well.[20]

The use of such drugs in aversion therapy has to some extent been replaced by electric shock within the past five years. The rationale for this change in technique is not based on proven differences in the therapeutic effectiveness of electric shock over drugs to provide the aversive stimulus. Rather, the change is justified on the basis of the convenience and control offered by shock administration, and the apparent efficacy of electric shock as an aversive stimulus in animal experimentation.[21] In view of the recent work of Garcia and Koelling[22] and Rogin, [23] where nausea-inducing drugs were administered to animals to elicit profound taste aversions, it would be worthwhile to reconsider the use of these agents in aversion conditioning in man, particularly in alcohol aversion conditioning.

**2. Therapeutic adjuvants.** Brady,[24] Friedman, [25,26] and Friedman and Silverstone[27] have used intravenous barbiturate to facilitate relaxation training in the systematic desensitization of patients with frigidity, impotence, phobias, and other conditions. A short-acting barbiturate (methahexitone sodium) is injected intravenously in a 10% aqueous solution. Here the drug acts as a means of inducing prompt, involuntary and profound relaxation in the patient. The drug is felt to facilitate relaxation, which then allows the therapist to proceed quickly with the desensitization procedure without the usual prolonged period of relaxation training. The reported success with this technique is encouraging, but studies with placebo controls and alternative means of achieving relaxation rapidly (hypnosis?) will be required in order to ascertain whether the drug is indeed a critical—or the most efficacious—adjuvant for this purpose.

The technique has received some inappropriate criticism based on animal experimentation with barbiturates. Various animal studies have shown that, in many instances, tasks learned while in a drugged state cannot be retrieved from memory when testing is carried out in a nondrugged state. Conversely, learning achieved in the normal state is frequently unavailable to the same animal while under the influence of drugs. This phenomenon has been labeled state-dependent or "dissociated learning.[28-30] The criticism leveled against the use of barbiturates in relaxation training is based on the belief that the dissociation of learning seen in the animal experiment will appear in the human therapy situation as well—that is, desensitization acquired while in the drug-induced state of relaxation will not persist when the patient is no longer receiving drugs: It would be dissociated, since the learning involved is presumably state-dependent. Were this the case, the new learning acquired in relaxation training carried out under light barbiturate sedation would be ineffective if the patient were exposed to similar anxiety-provoking stimuli when not under barbiturate sedation. But, this is not the case. Empirically, dissociation has never been observed in human beings undergoing this type of relaxation training. The criticism persists, however, apparently uninfluenced by empirical experience.

It is unlikely that drug dissociation could ever apply in the human situation when psychopharmacological agents are used. Dissociation in the animal experiments has only been produced with drug dosages so high as to cause severe ataxia and semicoma in the experimental subjects. Clinically, therapeutic agents are not used at comparable dosage levels.

**3. General anxiety reduction.** Many behavior therapists use psychopharmacological agents in much the same way that other psychotherapists use them—to help the patient cope with severe anxiety while undergoing psychotherapy.[8,31] Here the use of drugs is aimed at reducing the patient's anxiety so that it does not interfere with therapy. Among the various agents recommended are barbiturates, opiates, minor tranquilizers, and major tranquilizers in small doses. When the patient's anxiety level is reduced, drug treatment is terminated.

Anxiety reduction in behavior therapy is justified by a perhaps specious appeal to the Yerkes-Dodson law,[32] which states that optimal learning (therapy) can occur only at optimum level of arousal. Presumably the behavior therapist equates "level of arousal" with "level of anxiety," then reads the law as follows: Optimal therapy can occur only at optimal anxiety levels (as described above). Conversely, if the level is too low, it must be elevated. Elevation of arousal or anxiety level has been effected in practice with amphetamine, specifically in the therapy of enuresis.[33]

In spite of the behavioristic justification of drug use to affect anxiety or arousal level, this usage has met with criticism from various behavior therapists who believe that drugs interfere with learning or that dissociation might occur if drugs are given. The latter criticism has just been dealt with; the former strikingly parallels the argument against drug use by other types of psychotherapists. This, however, is not a legitimate criticism but an appeal to ideology which obscures an empirical issue that remains to be tested.

**4. Sympton-specific drug use.** One model of combining drugs with behavior therapy requires that the drug be used to correct the psychophysiological deficit (seizure, ego defect) that has generated a maladaptive behavior pattern, while behavioral modification techniques are directed toward extinguishing or inhibiting the maladaptive behavior. This approach is predicated on the hypothesis that a given pathologic behavioral pattern is a function of an individual's adaptation to a particular psychophysiological defect. While behavioral training can be used to eradicate the maladaptive behavior, the generator must be dealt with as well, lest the pattern recur.

Obviously, this method of treatment can only be used where the generator is identifiable and will be amenable to pharmacological manipulation. One use of this technique has been made in the treatment of agoraphobics. In this case,[34] imipramine was used to block the panic attacks which generated the agoraphobia while assertive training and systematic desensitization were utilized to provide reexposure to the phobic situations during which the phobia underwent extinction. This model has also been utilized in the treatment of phobias with MAO inhibitors where the psychotherapy was not specifically behavioral.[35] Wolpe[8] also reports the successful relief of anxiety evoked in specific situations such as flying or public speaking, by intermittent administration of the minor tranquilizers, and he has used antidepressants such as tranylcypromine and phenelzine as adjuvants, based on the work of Sargent and Dally.[36] In another study, the successful treatment is reported of a severe hand-washing compulsion by systematic desensitization combined with a maintenance dose of imipramine, 150 mg per day. Medication was discontinued 2½ months after termination of desensitization treatment, when the patient was judged markedly improved, and at six-month follow-up she reported no reoccurrence of her compulsion.

## Controlled clinical trials

Even more than with other combinations of pharmacotherapy and psychotherapy, there is a paucity of well-designed controlled experiments combining a form of behavior therapy with pharmacotherapy. A recent Canadian pilot study provides some support for the efficacy of combining antidepressants—in this case phenelzine—with techniques of behavior therapy. In this study, subjects receiving standard behavior therapies (systematic desensitization, aversion conditioning, and "flooding") were compared with others receiving phenelzine plus brief psychotherapy or placebo plus brief psychotherapy. All the subjects in this specific experimental group treated with phenelzine plus brief psychotherapy fared worse than the subjects treated with behavior therapy and furthermore relapsed after discontinuation of the drug. However, the authors report in their discussion that in their general clinical experience, when the drug was used *in combination with* behavior therapy techniques, many patients did *not* relapse after discontinuation, and they add: "With the present state of knowledge it seems advantageous to add drug therapy to one of the behavior therapies."

In the treatment of psychosis, it seems plausible that drugs which reduce psychotic thinking and improve organization should facilitate behavioral conditioning, but there are no controlled clinical studies in this area. Clearly, extensive systematic research, involving human subjects, comparing the efficacy of behavior therapy techniques with and without concomitant pharmacotherapy, is imperative.

## Theoretical and methodological considerations

The theoretical and methodological problems revealed by any consideration of the immediate and long-range effects and efficacy of all these agents are much like those involved in the development of a sound and cogent therapeutic rationale for clinical psychopharmacology in general. As such, these problems are beyond the scope of this chapter, except insofar as they apply directly to the principal theoretical postulates used by behavior therapists to ground their claims of clinical efficacy. In this connection three critical questions arise:

1. Do the chemotherapeutic agents utilized by behavior therapists in fact facilitate the extinction of anxiety responses and/or maladaptive behavior patterns?

2. Do these agents facilitate the learning—on stimulus-response (S-R) paradigms—of new and presumably more adaptive responses and behavior patterns?

3. Does such learning—if in fact, it does occur—effectively *transfer* to the undrugged state, both during the process and at the termination of therapy?

The need for answers to these questions becomes particularly pressing in the light of the outcome claims of behavior therapists. Friedman,[25] for example, goes so far as to claim unequivocally that "the desensitization which takes place at the treatment session is generalized to the life situation," and that "all the cases responded well and were symptom-free at the end of treatment."

The relative paucity of adequate studies combining chemotherapeutics with behavior therapy might at first glance seem to reflect the attempt of proponents of this emergent therapy to define its own limits of effectiveness before confounding the broader picture with additional variables. However, this rationale cannot be supported on either clinical or experimental grounds. In scientific experiments, important variables are studied and controlled for, not ignored; and in clinical practice, chemotherapy has had too evident a success to allow for indifference[37] There are other constraints preventing the widespread systematic use of drugs in combination with behavioral techniques.

The first constraint originates in the behavioristic tradition from which behavior therapy is said to derive its theoretical basis.[8] The only legal currency in strict behaviorism is the observable response; experimental observations and inferences which are not directly definable in terms of this currency are not acceptable for study.[8] This stand militates against the use of mentalistic concepts such as emotion or introspection and discourages the use of the intervening variable or mediating hypothesis; these are seen as nonessential factors and therefore as unmarketable commodities in the system. Despite professed allegiance to this theoretical bias, some behavior therapists have engaged in black marketeering as indicated earlier, by using the forbidden currency in various denominations such as the patient's emotions, mental imagery, and other unobservable mentalistic phenomena. They have been duly admonished for this,[38] but the serious clinical limitations imposed by a strict behavioristic approach keep them from trading exclusively with the legal currency.

Although all behaviorists (e.g., Hull, Tolman) have not taken such an extreme position, currently the most prevalent behavioristic paradigm (i.e., Skinner's) fosters and demands an empty organismic approach in the analysis of clinical phenomena. All that is acceptable for the analysis of behavior is an accurate "objective" description of the environmental contingencies that can modify the rate at which the observed response or behavior is emitted. No attention is paid to the experientially significant, nonquantitative aspects of the events generating the behavior—that is, etiology. There is no concern about the adaptive role of a particular behavior pattern, and subjective mental events are simply not to be considered. Behavior, being the dependent variable in the experimentalist's equation, is seen as being a dependent causal consequent—the result of competing stimuli (internal and external) which control the individual.

Drugs can have only a very limited function in this empty, passive organism which serves such behaviorists as their theoretical and experimental model. Drugs can be a stimulus which the organism discriminates, or they can be a means whereby organismic states are manipulated to change the reinforcing value of environmental stimuli (e.g., drug-induced thirst makes water a potent reinforcer). Intraorganismic processes, by convention, do not exist or are not important. Therefore, drugs cannot be used to affect them. Pharmacotherapeutics, as it is understood in the field of medicine, cannot be readily integrated into a treatment regimen which denies the relevance of intervening psychophysiological processes. At best, drugs can be used here only as stimuli, or as adjuvants or facilitators for various learning programs.

The orthodox behavioristic approach, as mentioned earlier, is often overlooked in the clinical setting. Drugs are used and presumably will continue to be used in combination with behavior therapy. This is not unacceptable from a scientific standpoint. Data generated from within the behavioristic tradition itself are beginning to force its advocates to a realization that intraorganismic variables are significant and may necessitate a reconsideration of previously enunciated "laws of the analysis of behavior" even though they cannot be specified in terms of the system as it is now proposed.[39,40] Perhaps clinical observation in the behavioral therapy setting will speed along this much needed reappraisal.

Even if this theoretical problem is solved, there remains one further and perhaps more obdurate constraint to the development of techniques of combined drug and behavior therapy. This problem is a delicate and complicated one. Although some of the leaders in the field are physicians, the vast majority of clinicians and researchers exploring the use of behavioral techniques in psychotherapy are clinical psychologists, not physicians. By virtue of their professional training, they are frequently reluctant—and are not licensed—to use chemotherapeutic agents. Those who do wish to do so must therefore cooperate with a medically trained colleague.

This restriction need only be pointed out here, but it forces us to be aware of the practical, economic and professional problems it creates. It is useless for nonmedically trained therapists to ignore this problem by resorting to empty organismic behaviorism. Furthermore, solutions to the problem will not be uncovered by ill founded attacks on the medical model. Yet failure to solve it might well sterilize the future of behavior therapy.

Finally, it must be mentioned here that behavior therapy is not alone in grappling with problems just presented. These interprofessional issues probably lie at the heart of many so-called theoretical debates about the utility of chemotherapeutic agents in all fields of psychotherapy.

## Rigorous clinical trials needed

Behavior therapists make impressive claims for favorable clinical results, emphatically disavowing the occurrence of symptom substitution. Many dynamically oriented clinicians level the charge of superficiality at behavior therapists and demand further validation before accepting the results. Nevertheless, behavior therapy is grounded in a theory and uses a method of treatment which only the most dogmatically prejudiced psychotherapeutic practitioner could dismiss out of hand.

Few behavior therapists are strongly opposed to the use of psychotropic drugs along with their psychological techniques, rather, most tend to ignore them. The literature examined here, while somewhat inconclusive, and even contradictory in some respects, would seem to support the claims of those few behavior therapists who support the utility of chemothera-peutic agents as adjuvants to behavior modification tech-niques.

Certainly, work in psychophysiology such as that of Olds[41,42] Olds, Killam and Eiduson,[43] Olds and Milner[44] and Neal Miller,[45] to cite only a few studies, indicates separate though interacting systems of drive, reward and punishment, and definite pharmacologic specificities at various areas of di-encephalon, limbic system, neocortex and reticular activating system, strongly supporting the hypothesis that appropriate chemotherapy could be a highly potent tool in promoting constructive learning—and constructive extinction. More im-portant, however, is the urgent need for further rigorous clinical research in this area.

Given the present state of our knowledge and the manifold problems which beset the mental health worker, an eclectic, pragmatic and syncretistic attitude would seem to be the wisest approach.

## References

1. H.J. Eysenck. Psychoanalysis—Myth or Science? *Inquiry* 4 (1961): 1. Published by Universitetsforlaget, Oslo, Norway.
2. _____. BEHAVIOR THERAPY AND THE NEUROSES (Oxford, England: Pergamon Press, 1960).
3. T. Szasz. Behavior Therapy and Psychoanalysis *Medical Opinion & Review*, 1967.
4. J. Masserman. BEHAVIOR AND NEUROSIS (Chicago, Ill.: University of Chicago Press, 1943).
5. J. Dollard & N.E. Miller. PERSONALITY AND PSYCHOTHERAPY (New York: McGraw-Hill, 1950).
6. S. Rachman & J.D. Teasdale. "Aversion Therapy," in ASSESSMENT AND STATUS OF THE BEHAVIOR THERAPIES AND AS-SOCIATED DEVELOPMENTS, C.L. Franks, Ed. (New York: McGraw-Hill, 1968).
7. J. Wolpe. PSYCHOTHERAPY BY RECIPROCAL INHIBITION (Palo Alto: Stanford University Press, 1958).

8. _____. THE PRACTICE OF BEHAVIOR THERAPY (Oxford, England: Pergamon Press, 1969).
9. E. Jacobson. PROGRESSIVE RELAXATION (Chicago, Ill: University of Chicago Press, 1938).
10. A. Bandura. Psychotherapy as a Learning Process, *Psychological Bulletin* 58 (1961): 143.
11. J. Burchard & V. Tyler. The Modification of Delinquent Behavior through Operant Conditioning, *Behavior Research & Therapy* 2 (1965): 245.
12. T. Allyon & N. Azrin. TOKEN ECONOMY: A MOTIVATIONAL SYSTEM FOR THERAPY AND REHABILITATION (New York: Appleton-Century-Crofts, 1968).
13. S. Rachman. Studies in Desensitization. I: The Separate Effects of Relaxation and Densitization, *Behavior Research & Therapy* 3 (1965): 245.
14. A.A. Lazarus. The Results of Behavior Therapy in 126 Cases of Severe Neurosis, *Behavior Research & Therapy* 1 (1963): 69.
15. R.B. Sloane. Behavior Therapy and Psychotherapy: Integration or Disintegration, *American Journal of Psychotherapy* 23 (1969): 473.
16. A.A. Lazarus. Behavior Therapy and Graded Structure, *International Psychiatry Clinics* 6 (1969): 134.
17. J.P. Brady. Psychotherapy by a Combined Behavioral and Dynamic Approach, *Comprehensive Psychiatry* 9 (1968): 536.
18. _____. "Drugs in Behavior Therapy," in PSYCHOPHARMACOLOGY A REVIEW OF PROGRESS. 1957-1967, D.H. Efron, Ed., PHS Pub. No. 1836 (Washington, D.C.: U.S. Govt. Ptg. Ofc., 1968), page 271.
19. C.M. Franks. Conditioning and Conditioned Aversion Therapies in the Treatment of the Alcoholic, *International Journal of the Addictions* 1 (1966): 61.
20. S. Rachman & J. Teasdale. AVERSION THERAPY AND BEHAVIOR DISORDERS (London, England: Routledge & Kegan, 1969).
21. S. Rachman. Aversion Therapy: Chemical or Electrical, *Behavior Research & Therapy* 2 (1965): 289.
22. J. Garcia & R.A. Koelling. A Comparison of Aversions Induced by X-rays, Toxins, and Drugs in the Rat, *Radiation Research Supplement* 7 (1967): 439.

23. P. Rogin. Central or Peripheral Mediation of Learning with Long CS-US Intervals in the Feeding System, *Journal of Comparative & Physiological Psychology* 67 (1969): 421.

24. J.P. Brady. Brevital—Relaxation Treatment of Frigidity, *Behavioral Research & Therapy* 4 (1966): 71.

25. D.E. Friedman. "A New Technique for Desensitization," in PROGRESS IN BEHAVIOR THERAPY, H. Freeman, Ed. (Bristol, England: John Wright, 1968), pp. 44-50.

26. _____. The Treatment of Impotence by Brevital Relaxation Therapy, *Behavior Research & Therapy* 6 (1968): 257.

27. D.E. Friedman & J.T. Silverstone. Treatment of Phobic Patients by Systematic Desensitization, *Lancet* 1 (1967): 470.

28. D. Overton. State-Dependent or "Dissociated" Learning Produced with Pentobarbital *Journal of Comparative Physiological Psychology* 57 (1964): 3.

29. N.E. Miller. Some Recent Studies of Conflict Behavior and Drugs, *American Psychologist* 16 (1961): 12.

30. _____. Some Animal Experiments Pertinent to the Problem of Combining Psychotherapy with Drug Therapy, *Comprehensive Psychiatry* 7 (1966): 1.

31. B. Blackwell. The Use of Tranquilizers in General Practice, *Prescribers Journal* 9 (1969): 29.

32. T. Silverstone. The Use of Drugs in Behavior Therapy, *Behavior Therapy* 1 (1970): 485.

33. G. C. Young & R.K. Turner. C.N.S. Stimulant Drugs and Conditioning Treatment of Nocturnal Enuresis, *Behavior Research & Therapy* 3 (1965): 93.

34. J.S. Brandes. Unpublished observations.

35. D. Kelly, W. Guirguis, E. Frommer, N. Mitchell-Heggs & W. Sargent. Treatment of Phobic States with Anti-depressants, *British Journal of Psychiatry* 116 (1970): 387.

36. W. Sargent & P. Dally. The Treatment of Anxiety States by Antidepressant Drugs, *British Medical Journal* 1 (1962): 6.

37. D.F. Klein & J.M. Davis. DIAGNOSIS AND DRUG TREATMENT OF PSYCHIATRIC DISORDERS (Baltimore, Md.: Williams & Wilkins, 1969).

38. E.A. Locke. Is Behavior Therapy Behavioristic? *Psychological Bulletin* 76 (1971): 318.

39. K. Breland & M. Breland. The Misbehavior of Organism, *American Psychologist* 16 (1961): 681.
40. D.K. Williams & H. Williams. Auto-Maintenance in the Pigeon: Sustained Pecking Despite Contingent Non-Reinforcement, *Journal of Experimental Analysis of Behavior* 12 (1969): 511.
41. J. Olds. Self-Stimulation of the Brain Used as a Screening Method for Tranquilizing Drugs, *Science* 124 (1956): 265.
42. _____. Self-Stimulation of the Brain, *Science* 127 (1958): 315.
43. J. Olds, K.F. Killam & S. Eiduson. "Effects of Tranquilizers on Self-Stimulation of the Brain," in PSYCHOTROPIC DRUGS, Garattini & Ghetti, Eds. (Amsterdam: Elsevier, 1957).
44. J. Olds & P. Milner. Positive Reinforcement Produced by Electrical Stimulation of Septal Area and Other Regions of Rat Brain, *Journal of Comparative & Physiological Psychology* 47 (1954): 418.
45. N.E. Miller. Visceral Learning and Other Additional Facts Potentially Applicable to Psychotherapy, *International Psychiatry Clinics* 6 (1969): 294.

# 8

# RESEARCH DESIGN FOR COMBINED PHARMACOTHERAPY AND PSYCHOTHERAPY TRIALS

The practice of combining two psychiatric treatments usually reflects the therapist's dissatisfaction with either treatment administered alone, as well as the hope that the combination will yield greater benefit. This therapeutic maneuver often stems from the favorable experience of a few clinicians, sometimes a single clinician. The clinical observations of the new treatment course may generate pilot work, and if pilot results prove promising, may spark and give shape to systematic hypothesis-testing studies.

The clinical gains from combined treatments may reflect either an additive or an interactive treatment effect. In the additive model, each treatment has a therapeutic effect; both together induce a total effect equal to the sum of the simple effects. In the interactional model, the therapeutic benefit of the combined treatments differs from (hopefully exceeds) the sum of the simple treatment effects, or is qualitatively distinct from the uncombined simple effects.

The most dramatic illustration of an interactive effect would occur where each treatment alone was ineffective, but the combination produced improvement. This situation is not altogether unlikely. In the treatment of agoraphobic patients, antidepressants have been reported useful in forestalling panic attacks. However, patients so medicated are frequently left with severe anticipatory anxiety over the possibility of an impending panic and therefore still cannot leave the house on their own. On the other hand, when directive-supportive psychotherapy is attempted without the assistance of antidepressants, panic attacks often continue and the patient is unable to progress. Yet when antidepressants are combined with directive-supportive psychotherapy, agoraphobic patients often quickly regain the ability to travel alone. Thus, if traveling unaccompanied were the specified therapeutic goal, neither drugs nor psychotherapy alone could be considered successful treatments. In combination, however, they can be successful. A positive interactive effect may be most likely when each treatment component affects a different component of the disturbance but the ameliorative effect of either component alone is not sufficient for a new functional reorganization.

Studies of combined psychiatric and drug treatments are difficult to conduct, for they present special methodological problems. New problems of treatment interaction emerge, and measurement, control and practical problems are compounded, thereby increasing the chances of deviating from the original design and introducing error. In drug studies one must be keenly aware of the issue of patient compliance with the prescribed drug regimen, although strict regular attendance to a clinic schedule may not be crucial. By contrast, in psychotherapy the patient need not do any specific "homework" such as taking pills, but compliance with scheduled appointments is mandatory. Combining the two treatments necessitates eliciting compliance with both requirements, a situation perhaps more difficult to maintain than cooperation with either treatment alone.

The discussion that follows is calculated to identify and hopefully set forth broad guidelines for many of the practical and research considerations which affect the design and execution of studies in the area of combined psychotherapy and chemotherapy.

## Treatment goals

Whenever treatment is undertaken, targets are set and goals are formulated; when the treatment is the object of study, the goals should be specified with maximum explicitness. The targets may be chosen on the basis of the investigator's clinical impressions or hunches, his own more structured pilot investigation, or other investigators' reports. The treatment goals may encompass any aspect of psychopathology, whether observed or inferred, and may be classified roughly as (a) behavioral, (b) symptomatic, or (c) intrapsychic.

Certain axioms of research design are relevant to the selection of treatment targets:

*First,* the behaviors which the investigator thinks may be altered by treatment must be well represented among the patients under study. It is surprising how often this self-evident rule is disregarded in studies of treatment efficacy. Not infrequently, courses of psychiatric treatment are reported ineffective in reducing, say, aggression, among patients whose pretreatment symptomatology did not reveal pathological levels of aggression. Unless the targets selected are relevant to the clinical status of the patients in the sample, failure in detecting beneficial treatment effects is assured.

*Second,* the less variable a treatment effect, the more easily it is observed. Treatment effects may vary among different patients, and over time within individual patients. Effects are more accurately measurable when they are stable within the patient and free of idiosyncratic variation among patients. Although complete evenness of therapeutic effect is never attainable, there are relative degrees of variability.

*Third,* treatment effects are more easily detected when the initial clinical status of the patient is stable. It is easier to observe treatment impact when targets do not vary considerably or tend to deteriorate. In contrast, treatment effects are difficult to establish for targets such as impulsiveness or mood lability. Fluctuating, ever-changing symptoms necessitate close long-term observation prior to and during treatment and therefore present serious practical difficulties unless one studies standard deviations of mood over time.

*Fourth,* the more quickly a treatment effect appears, the easier it is to detect. Whenever possible, the investigator should anticipate the length of time each treatment will require for effect. This formulation, if made before initiation of the study, would prevent the selection of targets that demand lengthy unrealistic projects.

Germane to the issue of time-related changes is the issue of contingent goals or goals that change as treatment proceeds. In psychotherapy, there usually is a sequence of targets rather than a single final goal. Further, the attainment of a subsidiary goal may indicate a change in treatment tactics. This is not as clearly the case for chemotherapy as it is for psychotherapy, although analogous conditions may occur. For instance, the acute schizophrenic may initially require large doses of phenothiazines, followed by a progressively lower dosage to a prophylactic maintainance level, accompanied by the introduction of an antidepressant. Such complicated treatment sequences obviously multiply study difficulties and necessitate careful preplanning.

*Fifth,* in the study of combined treatments, the specification of treatment targets must take into consideration the fact that each treatment may have different targets. Care must be taken that the targets relevant to each treatment are isolated from the others and taken account of at outcome. The omission of one or more of the effects of one treatment may bias the results in favor of the treatment, all of whose effects were measured.

Criteria other than that of clinical change may also be relevant to the study of efficacy. For example, patients in different treatment regimens may vary with regard to attrition rate. Interactive effects may also influence attrition rates. Or it is possible that even if only one of the two treatment components is clinically beneficial, the other component may have enabled the patient to accept the beneficial one. Thus, it may well be that for certain groups of patients psychotherapy and drugs are no better than drugs alone, but that patients receiving both are more likely to continue to take their medication. In such situations, psychotherapy would be a vital adjunct to pharmacological treatment. The reverse could also be true. A drug's modification of emotional distress may allow psychotherapeutically engendered insights to occur or new adaptive mechanisms to be tried.

*Sixth*, treatment effectiveness is most easily detectable when it is well-defined and manifest in the overt behavior of the patient. Thus, treatments which have marked functional consequences and lead to a reorganization of the patient's entire adjustment will be most easily measured. For example, if a hospitalized acute schizophrenic patient's thought processes are normalized, one may expect that his social behavior on the ward will be affected, as well as his ability to plan and move in a sequential, organized manner. Such a change in a central determining defect has widespread functional consequences and is therefore relatively easy to detect.

The same cannot be said about other changes often attempted. For instance, one may have the quite legitimate goal of helping a competent but dissatisfied patient to increase his work enjoyment. In such a case, a successful treatment may not lead—or even be intended to lead—to manifest changes in functioning. Therefore, when treatment goals entail subtle subjective changes, one must rely either on detailed self-reports or on meticulous observations over a period of time sufficient to obtain objective, operationally definable behavioral manifestations of subjective change. Although in principle one may observe the external signs of internal changes, in practice it can be difficult or even impossible to do so. Various types of patient settings, such as day, night or full-time hospitals, and rehabilitative workshops, may make possible the necessary continuous, intensive and systematic observation of patient behavior over the long term. Unfortunately, among outpatient populations seen exclusively via office treatment, one must rely on patients' or informants' reports, or on inferences drawn from interview behavior.

## Measurement of treatment effects

To go back to our patient "successful but dissatisfied in his work," we might establish at initiation of treatment that on weekdays he has difficulty getting up in the morning, has no appetite for breakfast, feels irritable, and is easily provoked. Further, we might find that he has difficulty keeping staff working for him. The list of his interpersonal and other difficulties might be extended indefinitely. To quantify the observable manifestations of internal distress, one might assume that the difficulties enumerated are secondary to the patient's work dissatisfaction and devise specific measures of such secondary effects. However, rarely is there any wholly reliable empirical basis for ascertaining precisely which observable symptoms are in fact causally secondary to the hypothesized central problem. To complicate matters, secondary symptoms often gain functional autonomy, so that even the relief of their inciting cause may not result in apparent change. Thus, in the absence of empiricial data indicating specific causal sequences of difficulties, the investigator must rely on *a priori* clinical assumptions. In such a context, targets have to be varied and should cover the widest possible range to insure that the relevant symptoms are included.

Difficulties are encountered in this schema when treatment effects cannot be discerned. There is no way of being sure that the treatment was indeed ineffective, since the investigator may have failed to pay attention to the relevant behavioral cues. However, the burden of proof is properly on those who claim therapeutic effectiveness. As mentioned, a large number of treatment measures is the best protection against such a problem although this in turn creates other methodological problems such as the need for large samples.

This entire chapter is concerned with change measurement in a broad sense, and this section deals briefly with some obvious considerations of measurement. A great deal more needs to be said about statistical problems in studies of clinical change, which are treated elsewhere in the literature.[1-3] In quantifying the clinical targets, the measurements must obviously be tailored to the targets selected, and the more likely the target is to be behavioral in character, the simpler the measurement. Ideally, the measures selected should have prior validation in pilot work to insure their relevance to the psychopathology under study.

In studying psychotherapy, measurement accuracy for both patient report and therapist behavior can be greatly increased by the use of audiovisual recording apparatus or videotapes, which also makes the use of an independent assessment team a relatively simple matter. Evaluation of patient status by professionals not involved in the treatment process is particularly useful for the evaluation of psychotherapy effects, since the patient's and therapist's opinions of progress are not independent or necessarily valid. Further, audiovisual recordings may be replayed until expert consensus is achieved and the cues upon which clinical judgment is based are explicated accurately.[4,5]

Another issue concerns the use of instruments such as psychological tests, especially the so-called projective tests, which are not tailored to specific targets but seem to reflect important aspects of intrapsychic processes. Data obtained so far with projective methods, and with intelligence tests as well, indicate that these measures are not reliably sensitive to clinical change. Many psychological tests have face validity for various personality constructs, but assumed face validity is not sufficient to justify the use of an instrument for purposes of measuring change in a systematic research context. In fact the widespread uncritical acceptance of psychological test batteries as a legitimate tool in efficacy studies requires careful review. Certainly, studies relating test changes to clinical changes are conspicuously infrequent.

It is also common practice to combine intercorrelated discrete ratings into single, additive scores. Unfortunately, the assumption cannot be made that items intercorrelated at baseline necessarily change together. Therefore, unless there is empirical evidence that these items are correlated after treatment as well as before, grouping them may obscure change. A combined score may fail to show treatment effect, whereas some of the items which it subsumes may in fact be change-sensitive.[6]

## Nontreatment variables influencing outcome

In any study of experimental treatment, certain nontreatment factors influence outcome. A detailed discussion of this topic has appeared in a previous Group for the Advancement of Psychiatry publication.[1] The major considerations in therapy research are the patients studied and the experimental context. Sample attrition may also be an important factor in outcome; some discussion of this factor is therefore in order.

**Patient variables.** The most important concern in studying changes in psychopathology is homogeneity of sample. The more homogeneous the patients with regard to initial target symptomatology, the easier the detection of treatment effects. Ideally, the patient sample should also be homogeneous with regard to treatment reactivity, but this would require exact treatment-relevant diagnoses, which are still lacking in the diagnostic armamentarium. It must be stressed that there are as yet no fixed standards for sample homogeneity. Rather, the specification of homegeneity is a function of our state of knowledge regarding the dimensions of psychopathology relevant to treatment outcome.

The extent to which clinical state influences outcome is so great that the selection of relatively uniform patient populations is a *sine qua non* of acceptable hypothesis-testing research design in the study of treatment efficacy. Unfortunately, many studies utilize nosological groups only vaguely defined (e.g., "neurotics") and report no discernible treatment effects, without investigating the possibility that subgroups with specific treatment responses were obscured within the vaguely defined population. Such studies contribute little if anything to our knowledge of treatment efficacy.

In pilot studies, the retroactive categorization of patients by the variety of clinical treatment effects may yield a useful nosology in the absence of any known treatment-relevant method for grouping patients prior to treatment. In such studies, replication is necessary, to avoid the possibility that the categories developed were based on erroneous *ex post facto* deductions or on chance factors. When experimental treatments are studied, precise sample identification is of the utmost importance in order to identify clearly the population of patients to whom the results can be legitimately generalized.

Many other patient characteristics may affect outcome, including a diversity of objective and personality variables such as socioeconomic status, age, marital status, education, employment status. IQ, early developmental traits, chronicity, self concept, anxiety level, social values, and so on. To require a sample homogeneous for variables that may affect outcome, as well as homogeneous for treatment targets, would enormously increase the difficulty of gathering an adequate sample. Therefore, it is unrealistic to demand both target uniformity throughout a sample and exact matching between treatment conditions with regard to all outcome-relevant variables. Randomization of treatment assignment, however, should at least minimize initial differences among patients in the different treatment groups.

Ideally, these outcome-relevant patient factors should be identified prior to the study, so that preliminary tests may be performed to be sure that they do not by chance differ sharply in randomly assigned study groups (as an extreme example, suppose that the patients receiving the experimental treatment are all married and the control patients are all single). Further, the clear definition and objectification of patient characteristics that possibly affect outcome permits the use of covariance techniques to allow for random differences in group baselines (if the requirements of this model are met).

Thus, a reasonable scientific compromise is reached if patients are selected for study on the basis of their diagnosis as well as the targets selected, and are randomly assigned to treatment groups. Covariance analysis may then be used in the evaluation of treatment effects to allow for other factors which may affect outcome.

**Research context.** The context within which the research is being conducted may be an important contributing factor in outcome. Patients treated in an inpatient setting cannot be equated with otherwise similar outpatients unless it has been demonstrated that the effects of treatment are not vulnerable to this factor. Of the dimensions discussed which influence outcome, that of context is the easiest to control and define. Although in the case of an outpatient setting due account must be taken of external events that may be highly important, it usually poses no problem to have all study members observed under satisfactorily similar conditions. However, these conditions must be identified so that it is clear to whom the study results may be generalized.

**Attrition rates.** Dropout rates do not represent an independent study factor which affects outcome assessment; rather, they are probably directly related to various characteristics of patient, treatment and context. As mentioned, attrition rates can in themselves be a measure of outcome, but they present special problems, because often dissimilar patients leave different treatments during the course of the study period. In the end the residual treatment groups represent populations different from those covered at the start, thereby invalidating group comparisons of treatment effects.

The problem of attrition is especially important in the study of combined psychotherapy and chemotherapy. It is quite likely that patients who drop out of psychotherapy are not clinically similar to those who drop out of drug therapy. To avoid being left with disparate groups, some investigators have matched patient pairs in such a way that if one member of the pair drops out, the other is automatically excluded from statistical group comparisons. This matching technique is the most rigorous in insuring against bias from differential dropout rates but it "loses" information about differential treatment effects. There may also be analytic problems if dropouts are unevenly distributed. The investigator should also compare the various dropout and remaining groups' initial measures to cast light on the causality of dropping out or, for that matter, remaining. Finally, because attrition rates tend to rise with length of treatment, periodic treatment evaluations are desirable to maximize the utility of the original dwindling sample.

## Definition of treatment variables

Terms such as *drug therapy* and *psychotherapy* give a broad indication of the nature of the treatment but do not give necessary information regarding type, dosage, length or frequency of treatment, so that these factors should be carefully specified.

**Drug treatment.** Drug treatment is relatively easy to define, since the chemical compound and the prescribed dosage can be exactly stated. However, the dilemma in design concerns dosage—whether a flexible dosage, where the treating physician can prescribe as much or as little as he sees fit, is preferable to a fixed dosage, where the dose is identical for all patients. Both flexible and fixed dosage schedules have advantages and disadvantages. The assumption that optimum pharmacotherapeutic effect can be achieved by flexible dosage regulation is made in many double-blind studies. However, this practice often results in underdosage, for the therapist does not know what he is prescribing and may be reluctant to risk an overdose. Furthermore, the patient is often at his best with the therapist, who may tend to undertreat him on that account.

On the other hand, when a fixed dosage is set, usually some patients are undertreated while others are overtreated. A combination of both approaches is often feasible: A minimum meaningful dosage derived from pilot studies is set, and the doctor is left free to adjust the patient's dose above that minimum. A flexible dosage seems especially appropriate for long-term treatment courses, since a drug may have different effects over time. For instance, in the treatment of schizophrenia the amount of phenothiazinc necessary to reduce the florid psychosis may, if administered over too long a course, result in a state of apathy and lack of spontaneity. This undesirable clinical effect can be avoided by appropriate reduction of dose while still retaining the antipsychotic effects of the drug. Ideally in all pharmacotherapy, clinical response should be correlated with blood level of the drug rather than with the quantity administered, because considerable variation exists among individuals in absorption and clearance.[7,8]

**Psychotherapy.** A clear definition of psychotherapy is a much more complex matter. There are many different modes of psychotherapy. Besides theoretical and practical differences, factors such as the therapist's personal characteristics, training and experience are generally conceded to affect outcome, although to what extent and with what patients is not well-established. For example, under the term *experience* little attention is paid to the kind of experience, whether it has been with neurosis or schizophrenia, with inpatients or outpatients, with acute or chronic psychosis, with group or individual psychotherapy.

The difficulty in terms of study execution is that if one wishes to study therapist characteristics in relation to treatment outcome, a large number of therapists is required. Alternatively, one might use a small number of therapists, but many diverse types of patients.

Even if no explicit attempt is made to relate therapist characteristics to treatment efficacy, these characteristics and their possible effects on outcome must be taken into consideration; therefore, therapists must be randomly assigned to groups receiving psychotherapy alone and groups receiving psychotherapy plus drug treatment. There remains the thorny theoretical problem that the therapist traits which empirically correlate with treatment outcome may not be the actual operative variables, but may be secondary to underlying operative factors (this is also true of outcome-relevant patient characteristics).

The crucial dimensions of effective psychotherapy are as yet unclear. To provide objective definitions of psychotherapy, some form of case-time sampling techniques utilizing audiovisual methods may be necessary, since doctors' reports of therapy session proceedings may bear little resemblance to what is actually happening. Unfortunately, the use of audiovisual apparatus may in itself influence the therapist's and/or the patient's behavior. It seems doubtful, however, that a truly potent treatment effect would be vitiated by such interference. In fact, there is considerable anecdotal evidence available that such procedures are not deleterious to psychotherapy.

Most studies of combined psychotherapy and pharmacotherapy deal with the issue of treatment flexibility only for the drug but not for the psychotherapy. However, dosage is relevant to psychotherapy as well as chemotherapy, since frequency and length of visit are important aspects of treatment. Should all patients be on a "fixed dosage" of psychotherapy or, as with drug therapy, should intensity of treatment be variable so that each patient may receive what is felt to be for him an optimum "dose"? Our current knowledge of psychotherapy does not permit the construction of clearcut guidelines to the effect of "dosage" on outcome, and pilot work would be required for each concrete case.

The combination of drug and psychotherapy raises special problems, since the psychotherapeutic intervention may change as a result of the effects of the drug on the patient. This possibility is particularly relevant to the statistical analysis of the effects of combined treatments. When an analysis of variance is performed to determine the effect of each treatment independently and in interaction, it is usually assumed that one treatment does not affect the other. However, this is probably not a correct assumption in drug and psychotherapy combinations. If drugs are effective, they may affect patient-therapist communication patterns so that the therapist may engage in therapeutic maneuvers significantly different from those he would employ if the patient were drug drug-free.

For instance, patients receiving phenothiazines may have longer speech latencies and be relatively unspontaneous, thereby influencing the doctor toward a more directive and active role than he would otherwise assume. This clinical reciprocity between drug effect and psychotherapeutic maneuver emphasizes the advantage of audiovisual recording of the psychotherapeutic process. In this way, a comparison of the nature of the psychotherapy given the group receiving psychotherapy plus drug with that given the group receiving psychotherapy alone would be possible. If major differences were actually observed between the psychotherapeutic procedures for the two treatment groups, one question would still remain: Were differences in treatment effect at outcome due

to the drug or to the alterations in psychotherapeutic procedures under drug conditions?

## Questions answered by research design factors: The issue of controls

Since a previous Group for the Advancement of Psychiatry
report[2] details the issues of controls in psychiatric research,
this discussion is limited to certain practical and theoretical
considerations in the study of combined psychotherapy and
drugs. Obviously, the major variable that must be controlled is
the active treatment. It is standard procedure in drug studies
to assign patients randomly to matching placebos or active
agents in double-blind fashion. Placebo control is a simple
matter here, merely requiring similar packaging for the com-
pounds under investigation.

Another form of control is possible in pharmacotherapy
research. Whenever prior research has established that a
given drug is superior to placebo for certain patients, placebos
are no longer necessary in the search for more useful agents
for those patients. Instead, the therapeutically established
agent can be used as a standard against which other agents
can be compared.

In studies attempting to delineate the "active ingredients"
of the complex procedure known as psychotherapy, it is very
difficult to devise a "psychotherapy placebo" and to set up a
blind assessment situation. The mere omission of the treatment by which patients are randomly assigned to "no treatment" and are placed on a waiting list for psychotherapy is
rarely feasible, since patients desirous of receiving
psychotherapy are likely to drop out of a "no treatment"
condition and seek treatment elsewhere, thereby creating an
immediate attrition differential. Moreover, patients placed on
a waiting list may actually experience exacerbation of their
difficulties as a result of frustration.

Minimum contact therapy has been used to provide a comparison group for the usual form of individual psychotherapy. Patients come at relatively infrequent times for brief interviews during which the therapist does his best to do nothing. This "treatment" may provide a control for the fact of treatment and the arousing of expectations of help. Group comparisons would afford some answer to the question of the relationship between amount and kind of psychotherapy and the variety of therapeutic effectiveness. For instance, it is conceivable that to relieve certain forms of symptomatic distress, minimum contact therapy may be as good as intensive psychotherapy, both being superior to no treatment. On the other hand, for behavior modifications such as improved social functioning or sexual satisfaction, it is possible that only intensive or goal-directed psychotherapy would be efficacious.

Two other possible forms of psychotherapy placebos are random programed-answer therapy and absent-therapist therapy. In the one, the therapist gives preset verbal responses in a completely random, fixed pattern. In the other, the patient lies down or sits up and talks to a screen or tape recorder without a therapist present. Each method presents certain of the elements of psychotherapy while omitting what are usually considered the "active ingredients."

The notion of a single psychotherapy placebo should probably be abandoned, since psychotherapy is such a complex procedure. The more rational though difficult course is to attempt an hypothesis of the active ingredients in psychotherapy by constructing psychotherapeutic variations for comparison groups. For instance, one might test for the importance of interpretation of unconscious fantasy by developing a treatment employing all the usual devices except the interpretation of unconscious fantasy, and checking results of treatment with and without this ingredient.

There is no way of providing for a double-blind design in a

research study involving psychotherapy. The major reason for attempting to "blind" the therapist is to prevent his knowledge of the therapy from affecting his evaluation of the patient, and the closest approximation that can be made is to have the patient evaluated by someone who has no knowledge of the therapist's treatment procedures. An independent assessment calls for careful precautions that the patient will not reveal or give clues to what treatment he is receiving. Also, certain noninferential functional targets like job attendance, time spent at work, income, school attendance, marital status, etc., are impervious to rater bias and therefore offer tremendous measurement advantages.

A determination of the nature and number of experimental and comparison groups is a direct function of the research questions raised. The following situations are typical:

**Situation 1:** We have an experimentally well-established valuable drug treatment for a specified population with respect to a certain criterion. We wish to see whether, following suitable pilot work, a specified form of psychotherapy will either increase the degree of benefit for individual patients or enlarge the proportion of individuals helped. This situation might be typified by the research on combining psychotherapy with drugs for acute schizophrenia.

The design seems perfectly straighforward. Suitable patients are randomly assigned either to drug or to drug plus psychotherapy, with appropriate measurements made prior to and at the end of the treatment course, as was attempted in May's study. If an additive effect is found, this design will not necessarily indicate an "active ingredient" specific to the psychotherapy component. More seriously, the design will not reveal whether psychotherapy alone could have accomplished as much as psychotherapy plus drugs.

Presumably, pilot work done before formal experimentation could have indicated whether pure psychotherapy was a treatment method of the same order of possible efficacy as drugs. If this is considered likely, then a design encompassing three treatment conditions is indicated: (1) drug alone, (2) drug plus psychotherapy, and (3) psychotherapy alone.

If drug alone or psychotherapy alone works as well as drug plus psychotherapy, there is no necessity for combined treatment. However, if psychotherapy plus drug is superior to psychotherapy alone, it still remains obscure whether the superiority of combined treatment is due to the active effect of the drug or to the adjunctive placebo effect of receiving pills. To answer this question would require yet a fourth treatment group receiving psychotherapy and placebo.

Moreover, if combined drug plus psychotherapy were superior to drug alone, it would still not be clear what particular ingredient(s) of psychotherapy accounted for this superiority. Answer to this question would then require additional comparison groups in which drug treatment was combined with different modes of psychotherapeutic intervention. Similar considerations would obtain for the psychotherapy plus placebo treatments. Should psychotherapy plus placebo prove highly efficacious, the addition of comparison groups receiving placebo and differing techniques of psychotherapy would be required in order to ascertain the relative effectiveness of various psychotherapeutic methods.

**Situation 2:** We have an experimentally well-established drug treatment for a specified population that is valuable with respect to certain criteria but is ineffective for other criteria of the illness. Pilot work indicates that a specified adjunctive psychotherapy may lead to improvement in the drug-refractory aspects of the illness.

This situation parallels the first exactly. The only real difference is that the drug is considered effective on the basis of criteria other than the criterion under study, where its efficacy is nil. All other previous considerations concerning assessment of increase in treatment value apply exactly.

**Situation 3:** We have a treatment method which is only anecdotally attested to. Clinical reports indicate that its effectiveness might be amplified by combining it with another treatment whose value has not been empirically demonstrated. What should be done? Should we start with a multiple group study of each treatment, treatment combination, and non-treatment controls?

This Committee's moderate preference would be to start with studies of each treatment singly—to determine first whether the clinically attested value of the anecdotal method and the presumptive value of the proposed adjunctive treatment can be scientifically verified. This tends to be a great problem in most psychotherapy research, where systematic validation of long-term outcome is rarely attempted. However, a study that would seek to establish simulatneously both simple and complex treatment effects without any prior pilot work appears to be methodologically unsound and indeed perhaps unduly risky for the patients involved.

Superficially, this might seem to contradict the findings of the previously mentioned example of drug-psychotherapy interaction in the case of agoraphobia. In that case, with respect to the outcome criterion of independent travel, neither drug nor psychotherapy alone showed a wholly satisfactory ameliorative effect, but combined treatment did show it. If combined treatments were studied only when conclusively positive simple effects were previously found, then presumably this study would never have been done. The apparent contradiction is easily resolved, however, when one recalls that a simple drug effect had been found—that is, the drug blocked the occurrence of panic attacks. This effect laid the groundwork for adding psychotherapy treatment to allay concomitant anticipatory anxiety and thus promote independent travel.

It is also possible that a given drug treatment might manifest absolutely no valuable simple effects but still interact effectively with psychotherapy, as has been claimed for the psychedelic agents, but it would take extraordinarily persuasive pilot work to engender controlled studies of such an unpromising situation.

Analogously, psychotherapy alone may be a flat failure in the treatment of certain conditions yet may enable effective drug treatment to be maintained, thus producing an advantage for combined treatment. Presumably in this situation certain simple psychotherapeutic effects engendering patient compliance would have been manifest, so that one would not be investigating a totally unpromising procedure.

**Situation 4:** Instead of a separate control group, patients can be their own controls. Specifically, they may be given drug or placebo for a period of time and then switched to the other agent on a random, double-blind basis. This cross-over design can be repeated as many times as one wishes. Chassan[9] has called this method the "intensive design," since it provides for long-term observation of the same patient under varying treatment conditions. If a patient regularly does better on a drug than on placebo, this is a strong argument that the drug is beneficial for this patient. Chassan has argued for the advantages of using the intensive design with very few patients over using a design calling for large-group comparisons (i.e., extensive design). The intensive design does not of course obviate the need for specified samples from which generalizations can be made to the population at large. Repeated cross-over designs with larger patient groups may combine the advantages of both approaches, which are in no way mutually exclusive. In particular, such designs may help identify specific patient characteristics that are regularly associated with treatment success or failure.

However, the cross-over design poses certain measurement

problems. It is feasible only with short-acting treatments without prolonged carry-overs, a limitation which prevents its use in studies of many psychotropic agents, especially the phenothiazines and antidepressants. Also, cross-over studies are best done for clinical conditions that have a fairly marked fixity of symptomatology rather than a phasic course. Another limitation is that when studying the effects of combined psychotherapy and drug treatment, the only treatment modality which can be varied in a double-blind random fashion is the drug.

In the intensive design studies reported by Chassan, drugs and placebo alternate, while psychotherapy is maintained throughout the study period. It is conceivable, however, that patients could receive phases of psychotherapy on the cross-over model (e.g., 2 months of treatment and 2 months without). As with any form of psychotherapy, this phasic treatment could not be carried out on a double-blind basis, but patients could be assessed by "blind" evaluators. It might be argued on clinical grounds that psychotherapy is not a short-acting therapeutic intervention, yet there is little systematic evidence available on this point. It is highly probable that the carry-over effects of psychotherapy vary with the type of patient. Cross-over psychotherapy designs might provide some answers to this question. The undertaking of such research would probably be extremely difficult in the usual clinical facility, however, because the course of treatment involved is at marked variance with most clinicians' goals and procedures.

## References

1. Group for the Advancement of Psychiatry. PSYCHIATRIC RE-SEARCH AND THE ASSESSMENT OF CHANGE, Report No. 63 (New York: GAP, 1966).
2. _____. SOME OBSERVATIONS ON CONTROLS IN PSYCHIATRIC RESEARCH, Report No. 42 (New York: GAP, 1959).

3. D.F. Klein, S. Feldman & G.H. Honigfeld. "Can Univariate Measures of Drug Effect Reflect Clinical Descriptions of change?" in PSYCHOPHARMACOLOGY AND THE INDIVIDUAL PATIENT, J. R. Wittenborn, S.C. Goldberg & P.R.A. May, Eds. (New York: Raven Press, 1970).
4. D.F. Klein & T.A. Cleary. Platonic True Scores and Error in Psychiatric Rating Scales, *Psychiatry Bulletin* 68 (1967): 77.
5. L.A. Gottschalk & A.H. Auerbach. METHODS OF RESEARCH IN PSYCHOTHERAPY (New York: Appleton-Century-Crofts, 1966).
6. D.F. Klein & M. Fink. Multiple-Item Factors as Change Measures in Psychopharmacology, *Psychopharmacologia* 4 (1963): 43.
7. H.W. Elliott, L.A. Gottschalk & R. Uliana. Relationship of Plasma Meperidine Levels to Changes in Anxiety and Hostility, *Psychiatry* 15 (May-June 1974): 249-254.
8. L.A. Gottschalk, E.P. Noble, G.E. Stalzoff, D.E. Bates, C.G. Cable, R.L. Uliana & H. Birch. "Relationships of Chlordiazepoxide Blood Levels to Psychological and Biochemical Responses," in INTERNATIONAL SYMPOSIUM IN BENZODIAZEPINES, S. Garattini *et al*, Eds. (New York: Raven Press, 1973).
9. J.B. Chassan, RESEARCH DESIGN IN CLINICAL PSYCHOLOGY AND PSYCHIATRY (New York: Appleton-Century-Crofts, 1967).

# 9

## INSTITUTIONAL CONSTRAINTS IN THE STUDY OF COMBINED TREATMENTS

In reviewing the current state of knowledge underlying therapeutic practice in pharmacotherapy and psychotherapy, members of this Committee have repeatedly encountered the lamentable situation in which major public health decisions about education and treatment programs were being made on the basis of inadequate scientific data. Considering the magnitude of mental health problems, current efforts devoted to systematic evaluation of therapeutic modalities are insufficient in number and scope and are hindered by institutional and organizational structures at local and national levels. Committee members recognize that the issues raised in this chapter go beyond scientific methodology and clinical practice to involve major public policy, but we strongly believe that new approaches are required.

The obstacles to be considered in this discussion are those raised by conflicts of role definitions and by organizational constraints on the logistics of treatment and the accumulation of data. Psychiatric staffs often view research procedures as unrewarding nuisances. A number of reasons can be identified for this negative attitude toward research, which, for one thing, is a function of how psychiatrists perceive their role vis-a-vis their patients. With good reason, psychiatric staff may not be fully convinced of the efficacy of their therapeutic techniques, yet in order to justify their activities and their remuneration, they are compelled to make an ideological commitment to them. A covert anxiety about the real effectiveness of their treatments frequently renders them touchy,

163

and resentful of the procedures designed to assess the actual efficacy of their methods. Therefore, it is easy for them to stereotype the researcher as a snoop who from his ivory tower has never had to confront the manifold practical problems of patient care. Another consequence of their commitment to current psychiatric practices is the belief of many of them that patients in research programs are being deprived of effective treatment.

Professionals in general and psychiatrists in particular have derived marked ego gratification from the feeling of autonomy. As a result, they often find studies of treatment efficacy difficult to tolerate insofar as they are based on principles of design which prevent participating physicians from prescribing as they see fit. Among the procedures frequently required in objective treatment evaluations are placebo control, random assignment of patients to comparison groups, and double-blinding as to the nature of the therapeutic intervention under study. All these procedures are associated with negative feelings in the minds of many clinicians. In illustrations, placebo control groups are methodologically necessary when evaluating a situation where there is no established standard of treatment efficacy—a situation all too frequent in medicine and psychiatry. Nonetheless, most clinicians are reluctant to adopt a self-critical attitude and to accept the fact that many of their procedures have never been clearly demonstrated to be useful. In consequence, they resent placebo controls as a deprivation of needed treatment.

The idea of random assignment often provokes negative feelings in attending clinicians, who believe that they are best qualified to determine optimal treatment for the individual patient, and that they are being asked to play dice with patients by accepting random assignment procedures. Similarly, double-blind techniques arouse anxiety in the conscientious, protective psychiatric staff charged with the care of the patient who, while still responsible for his well-being, are at the same time kept ignorant of matters central to the patient's welfare. This problem is in part solved by the accepted practice of initial approval and periodic review of research procedures by human studies committees.

May has pointed out that however difficult the creation of a rigorous research design, this is a much simpler task than actually executing one. Courage and empathy, administrative expertise in obtaining cooperation from physicians, nurses and other staff, and an appropriate power base are essential for the enforcement of those controls crucial to the conduct of a rigorous experiment. Much clinical research has foundered not because of poor study design, but because of poor execution.

In addition to role conflicts of personnel, other obstacles to controlled evaluations of therapy are encountered in organizational constraints imposed by the present logistics of patient care. Scientific study of treatment efficacy demands large samples of patients with relatively homogeneous diagnoses, stages of illness, and treatment goals. Neither private practice nor clinics nor hospitals can provide such groups of patients. For the most part, even very large hospitals are large only from the point of view of serving many chronic patients. Therefore, culling a relatively homogeneous group of patients from the admissions of even a very large hospital is an extremely difficult matter.

When the Veterans Administration and the National Institute of Mental Health recently conducted large-scale studies of relatively common conditions such as acute nonchronic schizophrenia and depression, it was necessary to gather patients from several hospitals to obtain samples large enough for study purposes. In such multihospital studies, each hospital collects a partial sample and treats according to a common protocol. The results are pooled. Multihospital studies are extremely complex in their development, conduct and analysis, since they incur enormous methodological problems and risks of measurement error. They are the product of current administrative necessity rather than a scientific desirability. Nevertheless, they offer the only currently feasible approach to the acquisition of the data needed in studies of complex designs.

In summary, the manner in which patient care is currently organized presents formidable obstacles to the conduct of research and to the development of research questions and research personnel.

## Some recommendations

It is evident that the present-day organization of psychiatric facilities does not provide an adequate program of intensive continued patient care, thus preventing the execution of systematic studies which would answer many crucial clinical questions. The limitations in our knowledge of the effects of treatment will not be overcome by the development of new research designs or statistical methods. Rather, what is needed is the development of clinical contexts which would make well-designed longitudinal studies of large groups of clinically similar patients feasible. Until methods of intensive longitudinal care are developed that will be appropriate to chronic and periodic debilitating illness, it is unlikely that the necessary long-term studies will be successfully undertaken.

One is forcibly struck by the tremendous distance by which even very good existing clinical facilities fall short of these requirements. This distance can never be overcome by patch-work attempts to modify present clinical facilities in the directions indicated. Entirely new additions must be created that will be uncompromisingly directed toward the same goal: the development of programmatic research hospitals, outpatient facilities, and aftercare facilities. By programmatic is meant that each of these hospitals should be devoted to the study of combined treatment methods in a specific, nosologically defined area. Such combined treatment-research facilities are warranted by a great number of mental health problems of concern today. These include the acute and chronic schizophrenias, mania, depression, character disorders of adolescence and young adult life, drug abuse and drug addiction, as well as alcoholism, psychoneurosis, childhood discipline and delinquency problems, childhood psychosis, geriatric organic mental syndromes, functional somatic complaints, sexual inhibitions and deviations, mental retardation, psychophysiological disorders, specific learning disturbances, and the convulsive and subconvulsive disorders.

Each hospital should consist of the best clinical facilities possible given the present limited state of our knoweledge. These would include full hospitalization services of day and night hospitals, and services of aftercare clinics as well as outpatient and crisis intervention clinics. With the development of an appropriate referral-triage system, each large urban center could easily support at least one 200-bed hospital serving some of the nosological areas mentioned. These facilities would have the single goal of studying effective methods of treatment. In the process of doing such studies much valuable information of nosologic, prognostic and etiologic significance would be generated, but the central work of these centers would be the systematic comparison of various well-defined treatment methods, singly and in combination.

Each center would be officially termed a research hospital and it would be understood that all patients would be volunteering for care in such a hospital and therefore volunteering for assignment to a comparative treatment study. In acute schizophrenia, for example, where relatively well-established methods of treatment are available, the patient should understand that he would be enrolled in a relatively short-term experimental treatment study program, and that if this should not prove effective he would then receive the best standard treatment methods currently available. Furthermore, following treatment, the patient would be permanently enrolled in the hospital's aftercare facilities. In the planning for such a research facility, special care must be taken to provide for unique patient populations such as those represented by upper or lower socioeconomic groups or ethnic backgrounds.

Of course, all of this should be free, to indemnify the patient for contributing to society's knowledge. Besides, by eliminating any financial burden upon the patient or his family, such free care would help to insure the long-term follow-up necessary for adequate treatment evaluation. For illnesses such as schizophrenia, which despite our best efforts may run a deteriorating course, collaboration would be warranted. The research center for studies in acute schizophrenia should interdigitate with the research center for chronic schizophrenia so that patients may remain under continuous care and study.

For those conditions such as the chronic character disorders, for which there are very little hard data on treatment efficacy, the patient should be told that he will be entered into any of several long-term studies in progress. The patient would, of course, be free to withdraw from these studies at any time. The resultant dropout rate combined with terminal evaluation would be one measure of treatment efficacy. Systematic follow-up of all study patients would be standard procedure.

Let us suppose that these centers contained approximately 200 full-time inpatients with a 4-month average length of stay. Within 2 years a sample of 1,200 patients in each unit could be studied. Such a sample would allow quite complex factorially designed studies to be carried out that would answer in a relatively short time many unanswered questions about treatment combinations, necessary length of treatment, and the like. The cost of such programs would be considerable, but when one recognizes that in any case the community is often paying for the care of these patients, the actual cost increase is not staggering. Furthermore, when it is realized that such research centers would also serve as centers for the training of therapists, teachers and behavioral scientists, their value to the community becomes even more apparent.

It should be clear that only the federal and state governments have the resources to develop and fund such projects. The present federal project and program grant method of funding research has resulted in a wide range of excellent work. Small research hospital units containing approximately 20 beds have already been funded and some brilliant work, especially in the biochemical/metabolic area, has been done. We are not suggesting a dismantling of the current system of research-supported organization, but the development of a new complementary institutional structure. Nonetheless, the fact that only large-scale programs of comparative treatment study can answer our treatment questions must be squarely faced. A continuation of the present system will only assure our continued failure to arrive at the answers we need. In turn this will do nothing to relieve the staggering burden of providing less than ideal care for so many chronic patients.

We recognize that all administrative innovations create new problems in the effort to solve old ones. However, such new ventures seem clearly indicated and should not be forestalled for fear of the complications that will doubtless arise.

# 10

## SUMMARY

### Psychotherapy and pharmacotherapy today

Psychotherapy and pharmacotherapy coexist as major mental health "industries." Each is utilized by hundreds of thousands of patients and each has an economic cost approaching the billion dollar mark annually. Large numbers of patients receive both. Often the choice of treatment is based more upon the therapist's training, skills and preferences than upon clearly demonstrated effectiveness. Theoretical and empirical bridges relating the two forms of treatment and their possible interaction are lacking. Clinical research data from which these bridges might be constructed are inadequate.

In current practice, psychotropic drugs are commonly used for symptom relief, while psychotherapy is aimed at the resolution of intrapsychic or interpersonal conflicts or for reconditioning, behavioral shaping, or reeducation. Yet there is clear evidence that drugs do more than offer mere symptom relief. For example, lithium appears to alter CNS functioning in a manner which is crucial to the treatment of manic-depressive illness. Phenothiazines have specific antipsychotic effects, perhaps through their action on CNS dopaminergic receptors. The successful treatment of a psychotic state by drugs may still leave the patient with serious neurotic and social problems, but without resolution of the psychotic state these problems may be untouchable by psychotherapy.

For twenty years there has been a tendency to consider pharmacotherapy and psychotherapy as antagonistic or competitive. There are many reasons for this. Among the most

171

prominent are historical commitments to ideology; differences in theories of the etiology of mental illness; antiquated training which tends to perpetuate ignorance of the principles, values and limitations of each form of treatment; differences in treatment goals; and legal restrictions on the use of drugs by nonphysicians. The competition between psychotherapy and pharmacotherapy has been attenuated in recent years because young psychiatrists, trained in both areas, use both comfortably. But even here the conceptual and empirical justification for both types of treatment is tenuous and research data demonstrating interaction are sparse.

Psychiatrists and nonpsychiatric physicians frequently prescribe psychotropic drugs in an unthinking and unsystematic fashion without adequate follow-up, safeguards or awareness of the hazards of behavioral toxicity. These drugs are correctly used, underused, overused and misused.

Nonmedical mental health professionals, such as clinical psychologists and social workers, have had no training in the indications for psychotropic drugs and are legally restricted from using them. In consequence, they provide inappropriate treatment for many of their patient-clients. This is also true for many psychiatrists whose training did not include detailed instruction in the principles and practice of psychopharmacology. Thus, older psychoanalytically trained psychiatrists tend to view drugs with suspicion or alarm, while younger psychiatrists trained in both forms of treatment frequently combine them, but without an adequate rationale.

## Reviewing the literature

A careful review of the literature shows that there is no systematic evidence whatsoever that appropriate psychotropic agents, at appropriate dosages, interfere with the psychotherapy of schizophrenia, depression or neuroses. Statements to the contrary are editorial and opinionated and are clearly based upon ideological commitments. Evidence is never presented to support these views by those expressing them.

For schizophrenia, the literature reveals that (1) the major tranquilizers (e.g., phenothiazines, butyrophenones) are central for producing symptom remission and improving social effectiveness, and that (2) the value of insight or uncovering therapy as a sole treatment or as an adjunct is dubious. Nonetheless, studies of relapse rates and social effectiveness with treatment forms currently in use show that there is much room for improvement. New and better drugs along with new forms of psychotherapy or sociotherapy require study and development.

In depression, recent and preliminary data suggest that pharmacotherapy and psychotherapy affect different dimensions of the illness and have additive effects. Drugs affected mood and diminished relapse rates. Supportive psychotherapy improved communication with close family members, diminished interpersonal friction, and assisted in resolving marital conflicts. Many more careful studies employing different types of psychotherapy are needed. In the treatment of symptomatic neuroses no reported study has shown that psychotropic drugs interfere with psychotherapy. Conclusions based upon clinical evidence are split as to whether minor tranquilizers combined with psychotherapy are of value. Clearly, more studies carefully designed to test this question are needed. Such studies should preferably be double-blind. They must equally consider the frequency and nature of the psychotherapeutic component, as well as the choice of drugs, their dosages and their continuous or intermittent use during periods of crisis.

## Remedial instruction and training

Training in the principles and practice of psychopharmacology needs improvement at both the medical school and residency levels. Continuing postgraduate education is even more badly needed. Such training should not be limited exclusively to practical therapeutics but should encompass the biological substrates of behavior, the biochemical and neuro-physiological effects of psychotropic drugs, and their be-havioral consequences in both normal and psychopathologi-cal states. Above all, such training should minimize the con-cept of mind-body dualism by emphasizing that alterations in the biological substrate need have no detrimental effect and may indeed have beneficial effects upon mental functioning and psychotherapeutic transactions. Psychiatrists, during and after formal training, should be encouraged to read the re-search literature independently and to *think* about the prob-lems addressed, their implications, and possible avenues to-ward integration of concepts and procedures in their solution.

## Future research

Some senior psychotherapists believe that studies of the psychotherapy of both the neuroses and the psychoses have been conducted utilizing therapists of unproven ability, and that the unimpressive psychotherapeutic results reported are not relevant to their practice. It would seem that the burden of proof is upon these skeptics and that maintaining this nega-tive posture demands the conduct and reporting of appro-priate scientific investigations to substantiate it.

The proper study of combined treatments raises complex problems of measurement, design and control. These prob-lems are not insuperable but the difficulties involved are both administrative and scientific. Research strategies can be plan-ned and research should be conducted on the potential value or hazards of psychotropic drugs in supportive psycho-therapy, sociotherapy, psychoanalysis, insight-oriented psychotherapy, group and family therapy, and the behavior therapies. Such studies should be double-blind to avoid bias and to permit evaluations of both process and outcome. Such studies also require appropriate stratified random assignment procedures and adequate controlled aftercare observations. Data derived from such well-conducted studies should assist greatly in improving existing forms of therapy and in weeding out unnecessary procedures. In the long run results from such studies would also enrich and modify existing theories of etiology and pathogenesis.

Problems in random assignment and controlled aftercare are largely administrative. Unfortunately, such evaluative study is alien to the present organization of clinical health care delivery services. The accompanying difficulties could best be overcome by the development of large research-oriented treatment facilities supported and operated for the specific purpose of assessing efficacy of single treatment and efficacy of treatment combinations in defined patient samples.

While awaiting such developments, the professional personnel at all clinical facilities have the obligation of specifying their treatment goals and methods for attaining these goals, and of marshalling the clinical evidence available that makes their beliefs more or less plausible. The introduction of proper treatment studies in such clinical facilities may foster a desirable skepticism about the utility of existing treatments, while at the same time generating improved treatment and follow-up methods.